To Mr. Neil Bush

With warmest
personal
regards
and great honor
to have the opportunity
to know each other

Yong-Jian
Cindy

Dear Neil,
We are honored
by your interest,
and your friendship!
Trip

CURRENT TOPICS IN ATHEROSCLEROSIS RESEARCH

CURRENT TOPICS IN ATHEROSCLEROSIS RESEARCH

YONG J. GENG
EDITOR

Nova Biomedical Books
New York

For permission to use material from this book please contact us:
Telephone 631-231-7269; Fax 631-231-8175
Web Site: http://www.novapublishers.com

LIBRARY OF CONGRESS CATALOGING-IN-PUBLICATION DATA:

Current topics in atherosclerosis research / Yong J. Geng, editor.
p. cm.
Includes bibliographical references and index.
ISBN 1-59454-428-X
1. Atherosclerosis. I. Geng, Yong J.
[DNLM: 1. Arteriosclerosis WG 550 C9765 2005]
RC692.C88 2005
616.1'36--dc22 2005011405

Published by Nova Science Publishers, Inc. ✢ New York

Contents

PREFACE

Yong-Jian Geng
University of Texas Health Science Center at Houston

Atherosclerosis is one of the most common chronic diseases that affect daily life of any adults. This arterial disease remains as the number one cause of death and disability in countries with developed society. Atherosclerosis-related illness is also arising in developing countries with improved economy. Heart attack and stroke, two major life-threatening complications of atherosclerosis account for more than 50% total death in the developed society.

For many decades, scientists and clinicians have been working together to delineate the molecular and cellular basis of atherosclerosis and to develop new medicines to prevent and treat this disease. Indeed, new theories, drugs and interventions have been developed in the fight against atherosclerosis, leading to decline in the death rate of coronary heart disease. However, the prevalence of atherosclerosis remains high. We have been able to slow down the disease progression or make it regression, and yet to date, we have not been able to cure atherosclerosis. We have identified several major risk factors and clarified its epidemics, but not fully understood the pathogenesis of atherosclerosis.

The purpose of this new book is to provide an update of recent advances in the basic and clinical research on atherosclerosis as well as a forum on which basic scientists and clinicians presents their views on different aspects of atherogenesis, vascular injury and repair. We attempt to focus on the cellular and molecular mechanisms underlying the development of atherosclerosis, and provide novel ideas for medicinal interventions to prevent and treat this disease. The first part of this book covers the basic pathological features of atherosclerosis, and a wide scope of signaling molecules involved in vascular cell functions, while subsequent sections will be more thematic; dedicated to a specific metabolic areas or to specific pharmaceutical targets. Because inflammation and hypertension or kidney dysfunction contribute greatly to the development of atherosclerosis, several chapters will address inflammatory mediates, ion channel and kidney metabolisms.

The book is the result of collaborative efforts from different investigators with many years of experience in atherosclerosis research. I sincerely appreciate all the contributors for their hard working and collaboration. In particular, I thank Dr. James T. Willerson, Professor of Medicine and President of University of Texas Health Science Center at Houston, and Dr. Ferid Murad, Professor and Director, Institute of Molecular Medicine, University of Texas-Houston Medical School, 98' Nobel Price Laureate, for their encouragement and contribution to this book. Finally, I would like to thank Susanna Patras for her tireless work in putting all the works together, and all of my colleagues for their scientific discussion and suggestions.

INTRODUCTION

Yong-Jian Geng
University of Texas Health Science Center at Houston

BACKGROUND

Atherosclerosis is a chronic arterial disease that occurs in young age and causes disruption of blood supply to organs or tissues in adults, leading to ischemic injury. This disease serves as a major limiting factor for healthy life and longevity. Its clinical consequences are often life-threatening; it contributes to the development of heart attack and stroke, two most common causes of death in developed society. Atherosclerosis-related diseases are a leading cause of death and impairment in the United States, affecting over 60 million people. Additionally, 50% of Americans have elevated levels of cholesterol that place them at high risk for developing coronary artery disease. The high mortality of atherosclerosis, the widespread suffering, and the huge economic impact demand integrated scientific investigations, medical approaches and therapies.

Although the terms, atherosclerosis and arteriosclerosis, are used interchangeably, strictly speaking, arteriosclerosis (or "hardening of the arteries") is one type of atherosclerosis. Arteriosclerosis is actually a generic term for a number of diseases in which the arterial wall hardens and loses elasticity. The term atherosclerosis is derived from combining the Greek words athero (paste) and sclerosis (hardness). Atherosclerosis involves a process that causes a build-up of deposits on artery walls called plaque. Typically, the deposits occur in the tunica intima (the innermost layer of a blood vessel) of large and medium-sized arteries. The plaques contain fatty substances, cholesterol, cellular waste products, fibrin found in blood, and calcium. Plaque can grow large enough to block the flow of blood through an artery. A build-up of plaque or a rupture occurring within the plaque can result in a blood clot. The dislodged plaque material can travel to other parts of the body (e.g., brain, heart, kidneys, and legs), resulting in embolisms and subsequently injury to tissues and organs, principally by blocking blood flow through smaller arteries. Atherosclerosis is a progressive, complex disease often associated with the aging process, but for some it starts much earlier in life. Early signs of atherosclerosis may occur in children.[9] Half of the children and siblings of individuals with diseased coronary arteries had signs of atherosclerosis, even though they had no symptoms of heart or vessel disease.

Atherosclerosis is responsible for coronary heart disease (CHD), myocardial infarction (MI), angina pectoris, cerebral vascular disease (CVD), thrombotic stroke, transient ischemic attacks (TIAs), insufficient blood supply to lower limbs and feet (claudication), organ damage, and vascular complications of diabetes. Because symptoms can be few or minor in the early stages, atherosclerosis is referred to as "the silent killer" because it can progress undetected for years, particularly in individuals who are at high risk for heart disease. Epidemiological investigations have identified major risk factors for atherosclerosis, including hypercholesterolemia, hypertension, aging, smoking, diabetes, and obesity. These risk factors may contribute to atherogenesis individually or synergistically.

Color graphics are presented at the end of the introduction.

Atherosclerotic Lesions

The normal arterial wall has fine layers of endothelium, intima, media and adventitia (Fig.1). When atherosclerosis occurs, the structure of these layers is disrupted, characterized by the slow buildup of deposits of fatty substances (mainly cholesterol and its derivatives), tissue or cellular waste products, calcium, and fibrin (a clotting material in the blood) in the inside lining or intima of an artery (Fig. 2). The buildup that results (referred to as plaque) can partially or totally block the flow of blood through the artery. This can lead to the formation of a blood clot (thrombus) on the surface of the plaque. If either of these events occurs and blocks the entire artery, a heart attack or stroke may result. In pathology, the earliest visible lesions on the lumen of the arteries are the fatty streak. This lesion can be found in people aged 10, but increases in frequency up to the third decade. The lesions are distributed throughout the arterial tree, but display a predilection for arterial curvatures and branch orifices [1,2]. Fatty streaks appear yellow because of lipid deposition (cholesterol esters and free cholesterol), and are characterized by focal accumulation within the intima of smooth muscle cells, monocyte/macrophage and T lymphocytes. These cells have the ability to secrete chemotactic and growth factors, which are mitogenic to various cell types, leading to proliferation of endothelial cells, smooth muscle cells, and fibroblasts. These factors include platelet-derived growth factor (PDGF), fibroblast growth factor (FGF), interleukin-1 (IL-1), epidermal growth factor (EGF), and transforming growth factor-β (TGF-β) [3,4].Monocyte/macrophages in the lesions have been shown to secrete a variety of proteinase including collagenase, gelatinase, stromolysin and elastase, which are of particular significance in view of the fact that disruption of the internal and other elastic laminae of the arterial wall are considered to be among the early steps in atherogenesis leading to luminal compromise and /or aneurismal dilatation. [5]

Fibrous plaques characterize well-developed atherosclerosis. They have been considered to be the characteristic lesion of atherosclerosis. Lesions are yellow-white in appearance and protrude to varying degrees into the vascular lumen. The fibrous plaque is composed of abundant fibrous tissue with substantial numbers of smooth muscle cells and myofibroblasts, fewer foam cells and highly variable degree of intercellular as well as extracellular lipid accumulation. Variable amounts of collagen, elastic fibers and proteoglycans contribute to intimal thickening, together with smooth muscle cells proliferation and migration [6]. In well-advanced plaques, the accumulated smooth muscle cells, monocyte/macrophage foam cells, and intercellular substances within the intima take the form of a dome-shaped fibrous cap covering a deeper central core of necrotic cellular debris mixed with cholesterol ester-rich extracellular lipid [7].

Complicated lesions are fibrous plaques that have been altered by increased cellular necrosis, haemorrhage, calcific deposits, or erosions (desquamation) of the overlying endothelial surface and thrombus formation. The complicated lesion can result in the compromise of coronary perfusion as a result of partial or total arterial occlusion due to the marked luminal protrusion of the lesions itself or because of the superimposition of thrombus. The latter may also result in the occlusion of smaller coronary vessels distally following platelet shower embolization. Progression of central necrosis within the plaque and accumulation of its "gruel" are often associated with weakening of the arterial wall, possibly as a result of increased monocyte infiltration and release of proteolytic enzymes. This weakening may result in dissection within the wall, aneurysm, or plaque rupture followed by thrombus formation and/or embolization of fragments of the plaque to the distal arterial tree.

A new classification of human atherosclerosis lesions has been proposed by the American Heart Association, which correlates the clinical progression of atherosclerosis with the histological changes. This classification divides the process from fatty streak to complicated lesions into five clinical phases and six principal lesions [8].

PHASE ONE (CHRONICALLY DEVELOPING PHASE)

Phase one includes the precursor lesions, which are usually found early in the life. These are divided morphologically into three characteristics types. Type I and II lesions represent small lipid accumulation in the arterial intima, and type II includes those lesions generally referred to as fatty streaks. Type III represents the stage that links type II to advanced lesions. Types I and II are generally the only lesions present in children. In the early lesions, disruption of the intimal architecture is minimal or absent, and the media and adventitia are not affected. Lesions types I, II and III are considered as the silent precursors of possible future disease.

Type I lesions. Type I lesions are the initial histological changes in the human intima, characterized by small, isolated groups of macrophages, containing lipid droplets (macrophage foam cells) [9]. In that lesions, hemodynamic or mechanical or infectious and immnologiacal injuries make possible the adhesion of blood monocytes, and possibly other inflammatory cells including lymphocytes and neutrophils to the surface of the injured endothelial cells expressing specific adhesion molecules. These monocytes enter the subendothelial space into the depth of the intima, and transform into tissue macrophages. When low-density lipoprotein (LDL) is present within the arterial wall, as modified by oxidation, it is taken up rapidly by the macrophages, which will typically transform into lipid-accumulating foam cells.

Type II lesions. Macrophages and smooth muscle cells characterize type II lesions, where macrophages appear stratified in adjacent layers. This type includes fatty streaks. The lipids are present within cells and consist, primarily, of cholesterol esters (77%), cholesterol, and phospholipids. The principal cholesterol ester fatty acids are cholestryl oleate and cholestryl linoleate (35 and 26% of total cholesterol ester fatty acids, respectively). Type II lesions are usually obvious in human coronary arteries around puberty.

Type III lesions. These lesions consist primarily of smooth muscle cells surrounded by intracellular fibrils and lipids deposits. Type III lesions are transitional lesions between the early and advanced lesions (type IV). Because type IV are classified as "atheroma", type III lesions are considered as "preatheroma lesions". Many intimal smooth muscle cells may contain lipid droplets. At this stage a massive, confluent, well-delineated accumulation of extracellular lipid (a lipid core) has not yet developed.

Phase II Lesions (Advanced Lesions)

Atherosclerotic lesions are considered advanced when accumulation of lipids, cells and matrix components, including minerals, are associated with structural disorganization, repair and thickening of the intima as well as deformity of the arterial wall. Lesions considered advanced may narrow the arterial lumen, are visible by angiography, and may produce clinical manifestations. Such lesions are of great potential clinical significance even when the arterial lumen is not significantly narrowed because of the dramatic consequences that may result from sudden changes in lesion morphology. The advanced lesions consist of three principal histologic types: IV, V and VI. The phase II lesions include types IV and Va, which have a high lipid content, not necessarily stenotic but prone to rupture. In type IV lesions, the fibromuscular hyperplasia is confluent and characterized by extensive extracellular lipid. In type Va, the extracellular lipid forms a pool or core covered with a thin fibrous cap that separates it from the lumen. The lipid core is a dense accumulation of extracellular lipid occupying an extensive but well-defined region of the intima. Between the lipid core and the endothelial surface, particularly in the so-called "shoulder regions" of the lipid-rich intimal lesion, is a relatively abundance of monocyte/macrophages, as well as lymphocytes and mast cells.

Phase Three Lesions (Acute Phase)

This phase is characterized by fissure or rupture of type IV or V lesions resulting in the formation of lesions type VI, which is characterized by a monocclusive mural thrombus. The associated stenosis may be clinically silent or result in angina. Fibrous tissue proliferation associated with organization of the mural thrombus may result in progressive occlusion.

Phase Four Lesions (Thrombotic Phase)

Like phase three, the rupture of type IV or Va lesions produces type VI lesions. However, phase four is characterized by the formation of an occlusive thrombus leading to one of the acute coronary syndromes –acute myocardial infraction, unstable angina or sudden death. Type VI lesions are responsible for most of the morbidity and mortality of coronary atherosclerosis. Disruptions of the lesion surface include fissuration and ulcerations. Factors that may play a role in causing or facilitating intimal disruptions of these lesions include the presence of monocyte/macrophage type foam cells and other inflammatory cells, including lymphocytes and mast cells, the release of toxic substance and proteolytic enzymes by macrophage within the lesions, coronary spasm and shear stress.

Phase Five Lesions (Remodelling Phase)

This phase represents the process of tissue repair and healing after rupture and thrombosis, including the lesion types Vb and Vc, which develop when layers of fibrous tissue are added to the type IV or type VI lesion. Incorporation and fibrous organization of mural thrombi of type VI lesions, with or without changes in wall geometry of the lesion, result in a more severely stenotic fibrotic lesion characteristic of type V lesions. Development of type V lesions during phase 3 may worsen the angina or result in total coronary occlusion. In type V lesions, layers of smooth muscle cells and newly formed extracellular matrix are added to the abundance of macrophage foam cells. Most of the collagen-rich fibrous tissue is accumulated between the arterial lumen and the lipid core replacing existing proteoglycan-rich matrix. Newly formed capillaries are present at the borders of the lipid core nourishing the cellular elements of the growing advanced lesion. Lipids also accumulate in the adjacent media, and the medial smooth muscle cells may be disarranged or decreased in numbers.

Cellular Basis of Atherosclerosis

The development of atherosclerotic lesions is regulated perhaps through a complex interplay between genetic and environmental factors. When pro-atherogenic factors overwhelms the anti-atherogenic, atherosclerosis develops and progress. Conversely, when anti-atherogenic factors prevail, atherosclerosis recedes or regresses.

Atherogenesis

Atherogenic Insults
(hypercholesterolemia, hypertension, diabetes, aging, smoking, obesity, inflammation, etc)

↓

Endothelial Dysfunction

↓

Permeability Increase
Microthrombi

Adhesion Protein Expression
Chemoattraction

↓

Lipoprotein Deposition

Leukocyte Infiltration

↓

Macrophage Differentiation and Internalization of Lipids

↓

Smooth muscle cell migration and proliferation

↓

Extracellular Matrix Synthesis and Accumulation

↓

Plaque formation

Figure 3. Schematic presentation of the pathological course of atherogenesis.

During the development of atherosclerosis, there is a constant change in the cellularity of the arterial wall. Traditionally, this arterial disease was considered to mainly involve the intima. Now pathological alterations have been found in all the layers of the arterial wall, including the media and adventitia. At cellular levels, endothelial cells play a key role in atherogenesis (Fig. 3). In normal blood vessels, endothelium provides an anti-thrombogenic barrier between the blood stream and peripheral tissues. Any pathogenic stimulation causing endothelial dysfunction or damage can trigger atherosclerosis.

Endothelial cells in atherosclerotic arteries show many changes in morphology and metabolism, characterized by increased production of adhesion proteins, chemoattractive substances, and vasocontrictive factors, and by reduced expression of nitric oxide synthase and vasodilating lipid intermediates.

Smooth muscle cells are the most abundant cells in the arterial wall, which carry out the task of maintaining the vessel integrity and regulating blood pressure. During atherogenesis, smooth muscle cells may migrate from the media to the intima and transform from contractile type to synthetic type of cells. Exposed to various pro-atherogenic factors, smooth muscle cells respond by producing more extracellular matrix and replicating at accelerated speeds.

Infiltration of inflammatory cells also characterizes atherosclerotic lesions. Macrophages and lymphocytes (mainly T cells) [3] exist in unexpectedly high numbers in atherosclerotic lesions. Many of the inflammatory or more precisely immune cells are activated and elaborate cytokines and other proinflammatory factors, in particular in the lesions prone to rupture.

In the plaque tissue, infiltrating cells are exposed to an extremely harsh environment with abundant cytotoxic substances, such as oxidized lipoproteins and proinflammatory proteins. Therefore, vascular cells may undergo high rates of cell death via apoptosis or other mechanisms of cell death in the lesions. If there are no sufficient numbers of newly formed vascular cells to replace the dead ones, the arterial wall may become weakening and ultimately ruptured. On the other hand, in response to the injury, surrounding tissue cells proliferate, contributing to the intimal hyperplasia. The cells synthesize extracellular matrix [6] and produce growth factors. Tissue repair or remodelling is following. Thus, a changed balance between cell death and growth characterizes the alteration in cellularity of atherosclerosis.

Another landmark of atherosclerosis is the presence of lipid-laden foam cells throughout all the phases of the lesions. The majority of foam cells are derived from monocyte-macrophages, and to fewer extents, from smooth muscle cells or others, such as mast cells. The main molecular pathway leading to the formation of foam cells is through the scavenger receptor pathway. Various types of scavenger receptors are present in plaque tissues and they mediate recognition and uptake of cholesterol-rich lipoproteins and their transport. Reducing cholesterol deposition and foam cell formation constitutes the cellular basis for cholesterol lowering therapies of atherosclerosis.

Summary

Atherosclerosis presents a unique case of chronic inflammatory disease characterized by deregulated lipid metabolism, apoptosis and proliferation.[4] The long-lasting process of atherogenesis displays various phases of pathological development. Each of them has its own morphological and metabolic features associated closely with the clinic manifestations of the disease and its complications. The cellular basis of atherogenesis involves both vascular cells (endothelial cells and smooth muscle cells) and non-vascular cells, in particular immune cells (macrophages and T lymphocytes). These cells are exposed to a harsh microenvironment with increased oxidative stress, inflammation and lipid desposition. The vascular tissue response to injury in atherosclerosis is evidenced by constant tissue remodelling and foam cell formation, which is a hallmark of atherosclerotic lesions.[7]

References

[1] Flaherty JT, Ferrans VJ, Pierce JE, Carew TE, Fry DL. *Localizing factors in experimental atherosclerosis*. New York: Grune and Stratton; 1972.

[2] Flaherty JT, Pierce JE, Ferrans VJ, Patel DJ, Tucker WK, Fry DL. Endothelail nuclear protein in canine arterial tree with particular reference to hemodynamic events. *Circ Res*. 1972;30:23-33.

[3] Libby P, Hansonn GK. Involvement of the immune system in human atherogenesis. *Lab Invest.* 1991;64:5-15.

[4] Ross R. Atherosclerosis: an inflammatory disease. *N Engl J Med.* 1999;340:115-126.

[5] Anidjar S, Dobrin PB, Eichorst M, Graham GP, Chejfec G. Correlation to inflammatory infiltrate with the enlargement of experimental aortic aneurysms. *J Vasc Surg.* 1992;16:139-147.

[6] Wight TN. Proteoglycan in pathological conditions: atherosclerosis. *Fed Proc.* 1985;44:381-385.

[7] Stein O, Halperin G, Stein Y. Cholesterylster efflux from extracellular and cellular elements of the arterial wall: model systems in culture with cholesteryl linoleyl ether. *Arteriosclerosis.* 1986;6:70-78.

[8] Fuster V, Fallon JT, Nemerson Y. Coronary thrombosis. *Lancet.* 1996;348:S7-S9.

[9] Stary HC. Evolution and progression of atherosclerosis lesions in coronary rteries of children and young adults. *Arteriosclerosis.* 1989;9(suppl):I-19-I-32.

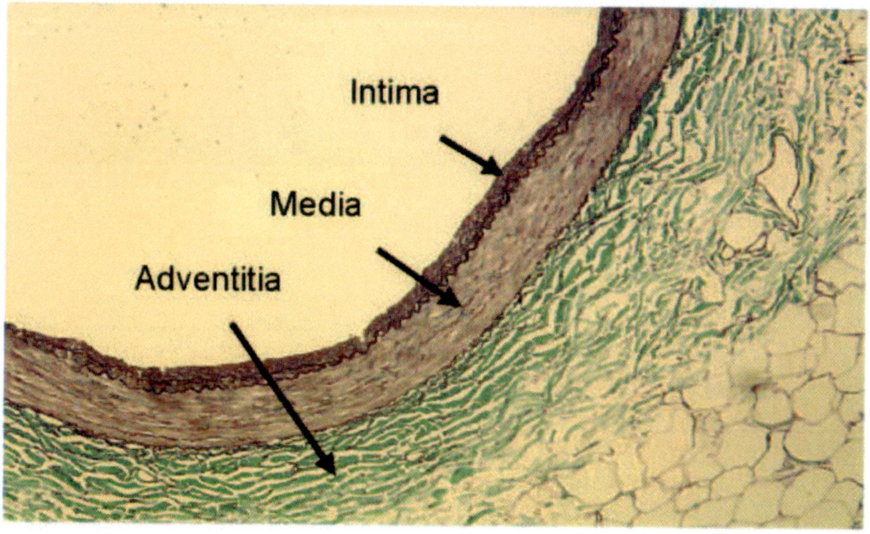

Figure 1. Normal human coronary artery. Cross-section of left coronary artery. Masson-Trichon staining. Image was taken by using x10 objective.

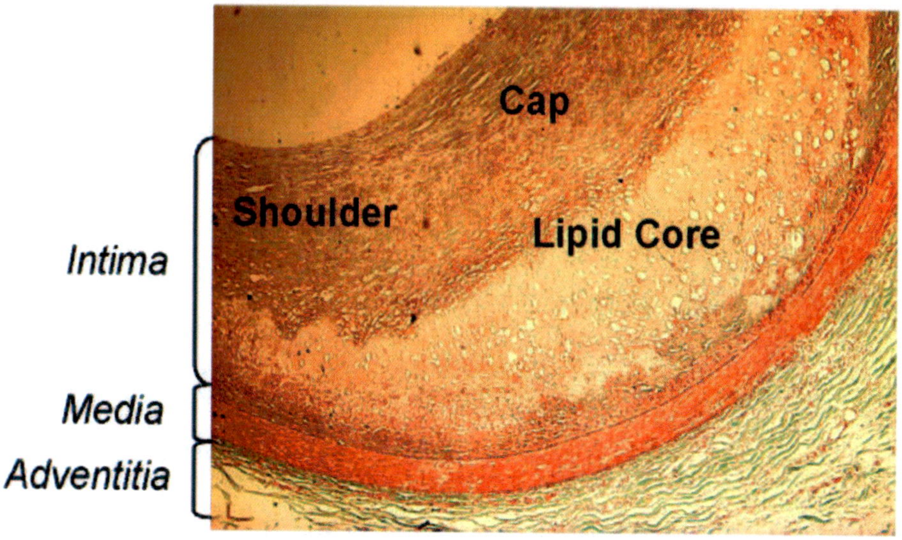

Figure 2. Human atherosclerotic coronary artery. Cross-section of left coronary artery. Immunostaining (red color) with anti-smooth muscle a-actin was developed by using the substrate Fast Red for akline phorsphatase. Image was taken by using x10 objective.

In: Current Topics in Atherosclerosis Research
Editor: Yong J. Geng, pp. 1-22

ISBN 1-59454-428-X

Chapter I

ATHEROSCLEROTIC VULNERABLE PLAQUES: PATHOPHYSIOLOGY AND DETECTION

***Mohammad Madjid*[1], *Silvio Litovsky*[2], *James T. Willerson*[1,2] *and S. Ward Casscells*[1,2,*]**

[1]University of Texas Health Science Center at Houston, and [2]Texas Heart Institute; St. Luke's Episcopal Hospital; Houston, Texas

ABSTRACT

Atherosclerosis patients develop life-threatening vascular syndromes including heart attach or stroke, largely due to disruption of silent, yet vulnerable plaques. Most recent series of studies on fatal myocardial infarction or sudden death due to coronary thrombosis have pointed to the underlying mechanism triggering rupture of plaques. Pathological investigations further illustrate the presence of significant amounts of lipids as well as high levels of inflammation in the ruptured or ruture-prone atherosclerotic plaques. Morphologic features of vulnerable plaques include a thinner cap, numerous activated T cells and macrophages, a pausity of smooth muscle cells, a lipid-rich necrotic core, eroded endothelium attached with microthrombi. In order to prevent plaque rupture and treat the vascular syndromes, it is important to detect or localize the plaques which are rupture-prone or vulnerable. Both invasive and non-invasive imaging technologies have been developed, and some of them are used in clinic. Primary and secondary preventation of atherosclerosis by eliminating the risk factors, hypercholesterolemia, hypertension, inflammation, and by changing life-styles have improve the arterial function and reduce the risk for plaque rupture. However, in spite of all the progress, scientists and clinicians still confront the challenge to promote regression of vulnerable plaques.

* Correspondence concerning this article should be addressed to Dr. S. Ward Casscells, The University of Texas Medical School at Houston 6431 Fannin Street, MSB 1.252, Houston, Texas 77030; E-mail: s.ward.casscells@uth.tmc.edu. Tel.: 713-500-6545; Fax: 713-500-6547.

Color graphics are presented at the end of the chapter.

Keywords: Artery, Atherosclerosis, Plaque rupture, Inflammation, Vascular image, Angioscopy, Thermoscopy, Nuclear medicine

INTRODUCTION

The age-specific mortality for coronary atherosclerosis has declined in recent decades [1] due to better control of blood pressure, reduction in cigarette smoking [1], coronary care units, early intervention by paramedics, increased use of aspirin [2], beta blockers [3], ACE inhibitors [4], statins [5-9], bypass surgery [10], stents [11,12], thrombolytic therapy [13] novel antiplatelet drugs [14,15], implanted defibrillators [16,17], external defibrillators [18] and other advances. [19]

Yet cardiovascular disease remains the leading cause of death in the United States and in other industrialized countries. Every year, approximately 1 million Americans suffer a sudden cardiac event (sudden cardiac death or acute coronary syndrome).

Many patients--and doctors--neglect primary or secondary prevention. Modifiable risk factors are not always identified and rectified. [20,21] Pressing problems include ignorance, neglect, denial, fatalism, lack of willpower, medication side effects and limitations which include aspirin-resistance [22] and the little-recognized late onset of statin efficacy. In the United States, obesity, [23,24] diabetes [25] and inactivity [26] are increasing, and stressful [27] factors are more prevalent, or at least established as risk factors and as triggers of cardiovascular events.

Studies over three decades have found that half the patients with sudden coronary death had no prior diagnosis of coronary atherosclerosis. [28,29] This was true in the Framingham Study, where participants were screened annually by a cardiologist, [30] and more recently in the Netherlands where, because of universal health coverage, there are no financial impediments to prompt diagnosis. [31] The reasons for the latter are complex, but the fact that myocardial infarctions are frequently caused by lesions with preexisting non-critical stenosis [32] is a significant component of this apparent paradox.

ATHEROSCLEROTIC VULNERABLE PLAQUES

Atherosclerosis is the primary mechanism responsible for coronary artery disease, ischemic strokes, and peripheral vascular disease. Luminal narrowing by inward-growing atherosclerotic plaques impedes the coronary flow and causes the ischemic manifestations of coronary heart disease. Acute coronary syndromes often develop following formation of an arterial thrombus and the concomitant dynamic vasoconstriction over an underlying disrupted plaque. The role of thrombi in unstable angina and myocardial infarction, proposed by John B. Herrick and others, was later verified through experimental studies in animals, and angiography and angioscopy studies in human subjects. [28,33-35]

Atherosclerosis develops as a result of injuries to the endothelium and arterial wall over a person's lifespan, beginning early in life. [36] In response to a variety of atherogenic factors (hypercholesterolemia, diabetes, cigarette smoking, hypertension, hyperhomocystinemia), endothelial cells express adhesion molecules and produce inflammatory cytokines and growth factors which recruit the inflammatory cells to the arterial wall. This inflammatory process involves complex specific cellular and molecular responses and reactions. [37]

Persistent injury, monocyte recruitment, macrophage infiltration, presence of activated T cells and mast cells aggravate the inflammatory state in the plaques. Plaque inflammation decreases the production of collagen by the smooth muscle cells and increases collagen breakdown through release of matrix metalloproteinases from macrophages and a simultaneous decrease in activity of proteinase inhibitors. [38-40] The sequence of events may lead to weakening of the fibrous cap and subsequent plaque rupture, or endothelium denudation that exposes the underlying highly-thrombogenic matrix and tissue factor to circulating platelets and white blood cells, hence initiating a cascade of events leading to thrombotic complications (Figure 1).

Sudden cardiac death and myocardial infarction develop at sites of plaque rupture or erosion, which are often associated with inflammation in the arterial wall. [41-47] The culprit, vulnerable plaques, account for up to 80% of acute coronary syndromes and usually demonstrate a large lipid pool (>40% plaque volume), a necrotic core, a thin fibrous cap (<65 μm), a large number of macrophages, outward remodeling, decreased collagen content of cap, and increased neoangiogenesis.

Willerson and his colleagues have suggested that changes in atherosclerotic plaques with consequent platelet adhesion and aggregation, release of thromboxane A2, and dynamic vasoconstriction lead to transition of stable lesions to unstable ones. [48,49] Several different platelet and non-platelet-derived mediators, including thromboxane A_2, serotonin, ADP, thrombin, oxygen-derived free radicals, platelet activating factor, and endothelin contribute to thrombosis formation and vasoconstriction in injured arteries. [49-53] (Figure 2). [54]

Most myocardial infarctions develop at sites that are less than 70% narrowed (% diameter stenosis). This was not fully appreciated for several years because of incomplete thrombolysis and intra-plaque hemorrhage, but studies of patients who had had a prior angiogram showed that half the infarctions arose at sites that had been angiographically normal, even though the vast majority of these patients had two- or three-vessel disease. [32] About two thirds of myocardial infarctions occur in atherosclerotic arteries with nonobstructive lesions without hemodynamical significance [32, 55-58]. In 50-60% of MIs, plaque fissuring and ulceration occur in coronary arteries with less than 50% luminal diameter narrowing.[59]

VULNERABLE PLAQUE: PATHOLOGICAL STUDIES

In the 1800s, Virchow [60] and von Rokitansky [61] debated the roles of inflammation and thrombosis in the pathogenesis of atherosclerosis. By 1928, Herrick had recognized the importance of coronary thrombosis as the cause of MI and sudden cardiac death. [62] In 1931, Olcott [63] described plaque rupture, followed by Leary [64] (1934) who described "rupture of atheromatous abscess" and Wartman (1938) [65] who described "rupture-induced occlusion". Clinical correlations were detailed by Schlesinger and Blumgart, [66] Chapman [67], Friedman [41] and Constantinides [46].

Our overview of 24 autopsy studies strongly suggests that occlusive thrombosis is found in 70 - 100% of fatal ST-elevation MIs, particularly 12 to 24 hours after the onset of symptoms. Thrombosis occurs in only about half of the victims of sudden cardiac death who die within an hour of the onset of symptoms and in less than 30% of those who have no symptoms prior to sudden cardiac death. The incidence of coronary thrombosis in patients with fatal non-Q-wave infarction or fatal angina pectoris varies widely between series.

Most recent series of fatal MI or sudden death due to coronary thrombosis describe an underlying ruptured or eroded plaque and an additional one, and occasionally two, vulnerable plaques, many of which exhibit rupture, often with luminal--and occasionally with occlusive--thrombosis. The vast majority of these patients have two- or three-vessel coronary atherosclerosis, and the majority of thrombi are found on plaques with more than 70% diameter stenosis. However, the large and well-studied series by Farb [68] and Burke [69] found the majority of fatal thrombi at sites less than 50% stenosed; most of the other victims had severe stenoses without thrombosis, and more than half of these had an old MI.

The most commonly described histology is plaque rupture with occlusive thrombosis. Typically, the ruptured plaque is large; but, after excluding expansion due to fresh hemorrhage into the plaque, the percent area stenosis is only 70 - 90%, corresponding to 50 - 70% diameter stenosis. The atheroma is typically large and characterized by a large necrotic core of lipids (including foam cells and cholesterol crystals) and unidentifiable debris, often with regions of old hyalinized hemorrhage and foci of calcification and angiogenesis. The fibrous cap is usually less than 65 μm in thickness and nearly devoid of smooth muscle cells (the cells which synthesize the collagen and the extracellular matrix proteoglycans). [70] The majority of such plaques exhibit foci of macrophages (often with a smaller number of T cells and mast cells) typically situated at the "shoulder" of the plaque. [71] Neutrophils are rare, except in recently injured plaques.

Virmani and colleagues have noted, in victims of sudden cardiac death and MI, that about a third of the fatal coronary thrombi overlie a non-ruptured but eroded (de-endothelialized and often ulcerated) plaque. [47] Approximately half have superficial infiltrates of macrophages as part of a healing response to the loss of endothelium (possibly due to infection, cigarette smoking, oxidized LDL cholesterol, trauma and/or senescence). Inflammatory cells and their cytokines and oxidants may also cause necrosis or apoptosis of endothelial cells. The noninflamed but denuded, thrombosed plaques often exhibit foci of proliferating or activated smooth muscle cells and immature extracellular matrix. Many plaques, including most that have an occlusive thrombus, also exhibit foci of intraplaque hemorrhage and thrombosis. Often, there is an old, partially fibrosed and partially hyalinized or calcified region whose thrombotic origin is likely because it can be stained with antibodies against fibrin. [72,73] These features suggest that plaques can grow episodically, due to thrombosis with incomplete lysis, followed by re-endothelialization.

The vulnerability of individuals to develop a coronary event is also affected by the status of their coagulation system. Vulnerable plaques and even ruptured plaques may be found in people with no symptoms prior to their MI. A rupture may occur at a time when the patient's blood is less prone to coagulation. Coagulation can be affected by genetic differences, diet, smoking, homocyteine levels, viscosity, and use of different medications. Local factors such as spasm, stenosis, proximal location of the lesion and shear stress may affect thrombosis propensity as well.

DETECTION OF VULNERABLE PLAQUE

Invasive Methods

Angiographic Plaque Assessment

Angiography has been the method of choice for assessment of the luminal stenosis in coronary lesions. However, it has limited spatial resolution, such that it is difficult to detect fine calcification, and fine irregularities of the luminal surface, including fissuring and superficial thrombosis. Most importantly, however, angiography--by virtue of its reliance on luminal contrast--reveals nothing about the plaque contents and thus, using current equipment and technique, angiographers are not able to assess plaque inflammation, cap thickness, or the size of the lipid pool.

In 1988, studies by Ambrose et al., Little et al., and Hackett et al. surprised angiographers with the finding that, in patients who happened to have had a coronary angiogram one to two years prior to their myocardial infarction, almost all of the thrombotic occlusions occurred at sites that had previously been normal or "nonsignificantly" stenosed. [32,55,56] Since then, four additional studies [57,58,74,75] have confirmed this. An unweighted averaging of studies of patients who had a prior angiogram (an average two years prior to infarction) reveals the following: 89% of the infarctions occurred at a site that previously conferred less than 70% stenosis and 60% occurred at a site that previously conferred a stenosis of less than 50%. The latter would be very unlikely to cause ischemia on a stress test unless they were particularly long or numerous.

Indeed, a study by Naqvi, Shah and colleagues examined the perfusion imaging stress tests of patients who subsequently had nonfatal myocardial infarction. Only 60% of the infarcts developed in a territory that was ischemic on the prior study, which exceeds the 33% random expectation. [59] The fact that the predictive value of the stress test exceeded that of the angiographic series may be due to the fact that the perfusion defects reflected the effects of multiple plaques in a given vessel, increasing the cumulative chance that a plaque would rupture; i.e., a reversible perfusion defect may not just be a region likely to be ischemic, but may also indicate an artery with multiple plaques.

Angiographic Predictors of Plaque Progression

Angiographic prognosis of the individual lesion is, in general, difficult. [76-81] Many plaques progress episodically, due to episodes of thrombosis triggered by rupture, erosion (denudation), or occasionally by endothelial activation or inflammation. [82] But there is general agreement that very tight stenoses (greater than 90 or 95% DS) often occlude over a period of weeks or months (presumably because of low flow, which promotes thrombosis) and generally do so silently. [58, 76, 81, 83, 84] For example, in Shub's study of 237 lesions in 65 patients, 23 progressed to occlusion, but only four caused a myocardial infarction. [81]

It also appears that a few stenoses spontaneously regress, particularly the more severe lesions, presumably as a result of thrombolysis and/or relaxation of dynamic vasoconstriction. [57, 76, 81] Regression is more likely in patients on statins and other lipid-lowering agents, and animal studies indicate that treatment converts lipid-rich atheromas into fibrotic plaques. [85, 86]

Progression from angiographically normal to total occlusion is generally a two-step process. [76] The majority of total occlusions were normal or only mildly stenosed on the previous angiogram. There are several examples: A. Moise found that 72% had been less than 75% DS; [87] J.I. Haft found that 80% had been less than 70% stenosed and 75% had been less than 50% stenosed; [76] R.N. Singh found that half the stenoses had been less than 50% at previous angiography; [88] B.G. Brown et al. found that 88% had been only mildly-to-moderately stenosed prior to occlusion; [89] and Alderman found that 63% of the lesions were less than 80% at the previous angiogram. [90] Thus, just as progression is not strongly predictive of events, angiographic severity is not a good predictor of total occlusion, or of MI.

To the extent that angiography is predictive at all, there have been attempts to identify angiographic features with prognostic significance. Numerous groups have studied complexity. Haft [76] and Freeman [91] found that angiographic evidence of thrombosis identified lesions that were more likely to progress over a few weeks to a few months. Davies found ulcerated lesions more likely to progress. [92] An irregular surface was a predictor of progression in studies by Haft [76] and Alderman, [90] but not by Davies, [93] and a long lesion was found to predict progression by Alderman but not by Joseph. [94] S. Ellis and colleagues found that the long lesion was predictive of progression only if it had an irregular surface. [95] In contrast, little or no risk of complexity was found by Guazzi, [96] Veen [83] or Ambrose. [97]

Spasm predicted progression in studies by Nobuyoshi [75] and Ozaki [98], but not in the study by Kaski. [99] Lesions in the right coronary artery (RCA) were more likely to progress, according to Nobuyoshi in 1991, [75] and Alderman [90]. Nobuyoshi also found that lesions in the LAD were prone to progress.

Ambrose found that proximal lesions were more likely to progress, and the location of the lesion at a branch point or on the inner curve of a vessel was also a predictor. [32] The attractive explanation is that the low shear (and perhaps the turbulence and increased residence time) induce expression of endothelial adhesion molecules and growth factors and promote both atherosclerotic plaque growth and thrombosis. [100-106]

Conversely, abnormally high shear rates can trigger thrombosis by activating platelets. [107, 108] Recently, Casscells et al. [109] found that clinical progression (over eight months) of "non-critical" lesions (that conferred < 50% DS) usually occurs at branch points, or at sites of calcification, or in plaques that transiently retain faint contrast after passage of the dye column (suggesting the hypothesis that plaque "blush" may reflect fissuring and/or revascularization, since newly formed vessels are leaky. [110-113] This is the first study to describe predictive progression in hemodynamically insignificant lesions, but the hypothesis needs to be tested in a longer prospective study. [109]

Angioscopy

Intracoronary angioscopy has been reported by numerous groups to be more sensitive than angiography or intravascular ultrasound in the detection of thrombosis and fissuring. Color patterns of plaques as detected by angioscopy have been correlated with different coronary events. Yellow, lipid-laden plaques -undetected by angiography- are more common in patients with acute myocardial infarction and unstable angina. These plaques often show surface irregularity and an intimal flap because of rupture or ulceration. In patients with old myocardial infarction and stable angina, smooth white lesions (presumed to be more fibrotic) are frequently observed. Angioscopy does not provide the deeper plaque characterization afforded by ultrasound and furthermore is limited by the need to inflate a proximal balloon to provide a blood-free visual field. This can create ischemia, limiting viewing time. More importantly, inflation in, for example, the proximal left anterior descending coronary artery precludes the evaluation of that critical segment. Nevertheless, angioscopy has provided important information about coronary syndromes and vulnerable plaque. [114, 115]

Combining the results of studies by Sherman, [116] Asakura, [117] Waxman, [118] DeFeyter, [119] Van Belle [12]0 and Mizuno [114] (unweighted averages), the culprit lesions in stable angina were yellow in 39% of cases, complex (including disrupted) in 28%, and thrombosed in 16%. In patients with unstable angina pectoris, the culprit plaque was yellow in 66%, complex in 53% and thrombosed in 56%. In myocardial infarction, 81% of culprit plaques were yellow and 42% were complex (an underestimate, since thrombosis- seen in 82%- precluded complete examination for yellow color in many cases).

Intravascular Thermography

Thermal heterogeneity of living carotid atherosclerotic plaques, examined ex vivo, was first described in 1996 by Casscells and Willerson (Figure 3). [121, 122] Stefanadis and colleagues described 26 patients with myocardial infarction in whom thermography revealed marked temperature heterogeneity. [123] All patients with unstable angina pectoris also exhibited temperature heterogeneity but to a lesser degree than those with MI. Among the 30 patients with stable angina pectoris, some had uniform temperatures like the patients without coronary disease, but a few had culprit plaques with lesions as warm as 0.2, 0.3 or even 0.5° C. above the reference temperature elsewhere in the vessel. [123] The temperature heterogeneity correlated not only with symptoms but also with serum levels of CRP and amyloid A. [124] In follow-up after angioplasty, temperature was a predictor of adverse events. [125] The mean temperature of the culprit plaque in patients with stable angina pectoris who had an adverse event in follow-up was 0.5° C., versus 0.1° C. in patients without an event. [125] Stefanadis and colleagues also showed that temperature heterogeneity is decreased by statin therapy. [126] These studies did not mention temperature heterogeneity at sites other than the culprit lesion scheduled for intervention.

Lesser degrees of temperature heterogeneity have been noted by Verheye et al. [127], Webster et al. [128], and Erbel et al., perhaps because many more of their patients were taking aspirin and/or statins and, in addition, their thermography techniques do not obstruct flow, whereas the larger thermistor used by Stefanadis often “wedges” the lesion. It should also be noted that blood flow can potentially attenuate the measured temperature heterogeneity over the atherosclerotic plaque.

Toutouzas et al. reported a good correlation between remodeling index (defined as the ratio of the external elastic membrane area at the lesion to that at the proximal site determined by intracoronary ultrasound) and temperature difference (DT) between the atherosclerotic plaque and the healthy vessel wall in patients with acute coronary syndromes [129]. They also showed that serum MMP-9 concentration is correlated with temperature difference in patients with acute coronary syndromes [130].

Verheye et al. examined the relation of clinical presentation to the number of warm lesions. On average, half of the patients with stable angina pectoris had a warm lesion, versus an average of one lesion per patient with unstable angina and two hot lesions per patients with MI. [127]

Verheye and associates have shown that temperature heterogeneity is determined by plaque composition and macrophage mass. They randomized 20 New Zealand rabbits to receive 6 months of either a normal diet (n=10) or a cholesterol-rich (0.3%) diet (n=10). At 6 months, 10 control rabbits and 5 hypercholesterolemic rabbits were euthanized, and the 5 remaining rabbits were put on a normal diet for 3 months. In the hypercholesterolemic rabbits, marked temperature heterogeneity (up to 1°C) was observed at sites of thick plaques with high macrophage content, but no temperature heterogeneity was seen in plaques with low macrophage content. Interestingly, in rabbits who received 3 months of a low-cholesterol diet, plaque thickness remained unchanged, but the macrophage content decreased significantly [131].

Thermography is currently in human clinical trials in New Zealand, Europe, Japan, and the United States. Human clinical trials will determine the safety, reproducibility, and clinical utility of this method. Once approved, it may be used to detect vulnerable plaques and to predict the risk of vulnerable lesions and vulnerable patients.

Intravascular Ultrasound (IVUS)

IVUS is better than angiography to quantify lumen area, plaque site remodeling, calcium (and, in some studies, areas of low density), and to identify plaque rupture and thrombosis. However, it is less sensitive than angioscopy in the identification of thrombosis. In IVUS studies, ruptured plaques are found in most patients with MI, in about half with unstable angina, and in a minority of patients with stable angina. Patients with MI or unstable angina are also likely to have a second vulnerable plaque, particularly in an artery with multiple remodeled plaques. [132] An important caveat is that, understandably, the best results are obtained at centers with great experience and enthusiasm for IVUS. Moreover, IVUS cannot distinguish caps thinner than approximately 0.4 mm, whereas pathologic studies indicate that almost all ruptured plaques are thinner than 0.075 mm.

Ge et al. used intravascular ultrasound (IVUS) to study 42 patients with unstable angina pectoris and 102 patients with stable angina pectoris. IVUS identified 29 ruptures (only a third of which were identified by angiography). No patient had more than one ruptured plaque. Of the 102 patients with stable angina pectoris, eight had a ruptured plaque. The disrupted plaques averaged 56% diameter stenosis versus 68% for the nondisrupted but symptomatic plaques. The disrupted plaques also had a thinner cap (0.47 ± 0.2 mm vs. 0.96 ± 0.94 mm), a larger echolucent area, and were more likely to be eccentric (94 vs. 64%).[133]

Of the patients with unstable angina, 21 exhibited rupture, one had an erosion, and 20 had neither.

In contrast, Rioufoul et al. found evidence of 50 coronary plaque ruptures in 24 patients with acute coronary syndromes studied by intravascular ultrasound. Seventy-one percent of these were in a nonculprit artery and 12.5% had ruptures in both nonculprit arteries. Only 37.5% of the presumed culprit stenoses were actually ruptured. Calcification was commonly found in the ruptured lesions and particularly in the culprit lesions. The subgroup of patients with ST-segment elevation infarction was slightly more likely to have ruptures than the patients with unstable angina or infarction with ST depression. [132] As found by Ge, angiography was not as sensitive as intravascular ultrasound in detecting rupture. [133]

IVUS Elastography

IVUS elastography technology is based on the differences in hardness and elasticity of tissues with different histopathologic composition. By measuring the local strain over the plaque, this technique can discriminate between soft and hard tissues. Elastography can assess the mechanical properties of the arterial wall as soft plaques have a higher strain level than hard plaques. Fibrous caps of vulnerable plaques have been shown to have a high strain level and elastography has been used for detection of plaques at risk of rupture. [134, 135]

Optical Coherence Tomography (OCT)

Optical Coherence Tomography (OCT) employs a laser (infrared) beam as the light source which is directed to and reflected back from the tissue. OCT measures the intensity of the reflected infrared light and has a remarkable resolution of about 20 μm [136, 137] Current techniques have a penetration depth of 1 to 2 mm. Studies have shown the ability of OCT in measuring the cap thickness and differentiating lipid tissue from water-based tissues. [136, 137] The major limitation with this technique is the need for proximal occlusion as presence of blood significantly reduces the OCT image quality.

Non-Invasive Imaging of Vulnerable Plaques

Computed Tomographic (CT) Imaging

Autopsy studies consistently demonstrate that calcification is a common complication of advanced atherosclerosis. More recently, multiple clinical studies have demonstrated that this calcification can be detected by fluoroscopy and - more accurately and quantitatively - by electron beam CT or multi-slice CT. [138] After normalizing for the age-related increase in arterial calcification, these techniques not only correlate with the extent of disease but also identify patients at risk of MI or death better than traditional risk factors. [139] Calcium scoring is not yet widely used in primary or secondary risk assessment, but it is useful to begin to ask whether this technique can be used not only to identify the person at risk but also the lesion at risk.

Specific features or combinations of features may be more predictive than a single score based on the number or density of calcium. Litovsky et al. have recently noted that large inflamed lesions typically have foci of angiogenesis and calcification at the periphery;

whereas, densely calcified lesions have little or no necrotic core inflammation or angiogenesis. [140] The large, mildly calcified and neovascularized lesion might well be identifiable by using contrast. Moreover, contrast with close inspection of cross-sectional images might reveal systolic dimpling or eccentricity indicative of a thin-capped, soft lesion. Contrast should also permit the identification of "plaque blush." [109]

A closer look at lesion anatomy and a follow-up study might well reveal that hypodense (lipid-rich) or heterogeneous (lesions which might have undergone previous rupture and/or remodeling) are at higher risk. It might also be hypothesized that lesions at branch points or in the proximal LAD or RCA, or soft lesions adjacent to fibrotic areas, are at higher risk.

Magnetic Resonance Imaging

High-resolution magnetic resonance imaging (MRI) is a promising method for non-invasive imaging of vulnerable plaques. MRI has been used for monitoring the progression and regression of atherosclerotic plaques over time and for visualization of arterial thrombi in vivo. [141, 142]

Magnetic resonance imaging is more time-consuming and expensive than computed tomography, and some patients are ineligible by virtue of pacemakers or other embedded metal, but it has extraordinary potential for plaque characterization. [143, 144] Moreover, spatial resolution can be improved with higher field strength magnets (e.g., 3T), surface coils, intracoronary antennae or superconductivity. Recently, several groups have reported that plaque macrophages can be imaged by their uptake of iron oxide. [145] Finally, tagging gadolinium or iron oxide particles with LDL or plaque-specific antibodies may permit molecular imaging.

Current Therapy of Vulnerable Plaque

Because there is not yet an accepted way to detect and follow the course of vulnerable plaques, there is no proven intervention for reducing the risk of plaque rupture, plaque erosion or plaque thrombosis per se. However, the risk factors for myocardial infarction and angina pectoris are nearly identical in most studies, and factors for sudden cardiac death are similar; risks of these outcomes have been reduced--albeit modestly--in most primary and secondary prevention studies by reducing blood pressure [146-148], cholesterol levels [5-9], cigarette smoking [149], and aspirin. [150] Some of the benefit is due to a slowing of atherogenesis and some to a stabilization of vulnerable plaque. A number of novel methods are under investigation to control inflammation at a local or systemic level to stabilize vulnerable plaques.

CONCLUSION

During the past two decades, we have witnessed considerable progress in understanding the pathogenesis of atherosclerosis and vulnerable plaques. Multiple methods are being investigated for detection of vulnerable plaques. A combination of several detection techniques may be used to screen and detect lesions invasively or non-invasively.

This can lead to development of more efficient methods to prevent and control coronary heart disease. A comprehensive preventive and therapeutic approach would considerably reduce the risk of fatal and non-fatal heart attacks.

References

[1] Hunink MG, Goldman L, Tosteson AN, Mittleman MA, Goldman PA, et al. The recent decline in mortality from coronary heart disease, 1980-1990. The effect of secular trends in risk factors and treatment. *JAMA* 1997; 277:535-42.

[2] Spencer FA, Santopinto JJ, Gore JM, Goldberg RJ, Fox KA, et al. Impact of aspirin on presentation and hospital outcomes in patients with acute coronary syndromes (The Global Registry of Acute Coronary Events [GRACE]). *Am J Cardiol* 2002; 90:1056-61.

[3] Waeber B, Brunner HR, Burnier M, Cohn JN. *Hypertention.* In: Cohn JN, ed. Cardiovascular Medicine: Churchill Livingstone, 2000:1518.

[4] Sleight P, Yusuf S, Pogue J, Tsuyuki R, Diaz R, Probstfield J. Blood-pressure reduction and cardiovascular risk in HOPE study. *Lancet* 2001; 358:2130-1.

[5] Sacks FM, Pfeffer MA, Moye LA, Rouleau JL, Rutherford JD, et al. The effect of pravastatin on coronary events after myocardial infarction in patients with average cholesterol levels. Cholesterol and Recurrent Events Trial investigators. *N Engl J Med* 1996; 335:1001-9.

[6] MRC/BHF Heart Protection Study of cholesterol lowering with simvastatin in 20,536 high-risk individuals: a randomised placebo-controlled trial. *Lancet* 2002; 360:7-22.

[7] Randomised trial of cholesterol lowering in 4444 patients with coronary heart disease: the Scandinavian Simvastatin Survival Study (4S). *Lancet* 1994; 344:1383-9.

[8] Downs JR, Clearfield M, Weis S, Whitney E, Shapiro DR, et al. Primary prevention of acute coronary events with lovastatin in men and women with average cholesterol levels: results of AFCAPS/TexCAPS. Air Force/Texas Coronary Atherosclerosis Prevention Study. *JAMA* 1998; 279:1615-22.

[9] Simes J, Furberg CD, Braunwald E, Davis BR, Ford I, et al. Effects of pravastatin on mortality in patients with and without coronary heart disease across a broad range of cholesterol levels. The Prospective Pravastatin Pooling project. *Eur Heart J* 2002; 23:207-15.

[10] Bradshaw PJ, Jamrozik K, Le M, Gilfillan I, Thompson PL. Mortality and recurrent cardiac events after coronary artery bypass graft: long term outcomes in a population study. *Heart* 2002; 88:488-94.

[11] Ashby DT, Dangas G, Mehran R, Lansky AJ, Narasimaiah R, et al. Comparison of clinical outcomes using stents versus no stents after percutaneous coronary intervention for proximal left anterior descending versus proximal right and left circumflex coronary arteries. *Am J Cardiol* 2002; 89:1162-6.

[12] Zhu MM, Feit A, Chadow H, Alam M, Kwan T, Clark LT. Primary stent implantation compared with primary balloon angioplasty for acute myocardial infarction: a meta-analysis of randomized clinical trials. *Am J Cardiol* 2001; 88:297-301.

[13] Holmes DR, Jr., Califf RM, Topol EJ. Lessons we have learned from the GUSTO trial. Global Utilization of Streptokinase and Tissue Plasminogen Activator for Occluded Arteries. *J Am Coll Cardiol* 1995; 25:10S-17S.

[14] Jarvis B, Simpson K. Clopidogrel: a review of its use in the prevention of atherothrombosis. *Drugs* 2000; 60:347-77.

[15] Yusuf S, Zhao F, Mehta SR, Chrolavicius S, Tognoni G, Fox KK. Effects of clopidogrel in addition to aspirin in patients with acute coronary syndromes without ST-segment elevation. *N Engl J Med* 2001; 345:494-502.

[16] Campbell RW. Postoperative arrhythmias and the role for implantable cardioverter-defibrillators. *Curr Opin Cardiol* 1993; 8:932-7.

[17] Chatrath R, Porter CB, Ackerman MJ. Role of transvenous implantable cardioverter-defibrillators in preventing sudden cardiac death in children, adolescents, and young adults. *Mayo Clin Proc* 2002; 77:226-31.

[18] Marenco JP, Wang PJ, Link MS, Homoud MK, Estes NA, 3rd. Improving survival from sudden cardiac arrest: the role of the automated external defibrillator. *JAMA* 2001; 285:1193-200.

[19] Park H, Safdar N, Schmidt H. Decline in mortality of coronary heart disease among whites and blacks in Wisconsin 1979-1998. *WMJ* 2002; 101:23-7.

[20] Hoerger TJ, Bala MV, Bray JW, Wilcosky TC, LaRosa J. Treatment patterns and distribution of low-density lipoprotein cholesterol levels in treatment-eligible United States adults. *Am J Cardiol* 1998; 82:61-5.

[21] Pearson TA, Laurora I, Chu H, Kafonek S. The lipid treatment assessment project (L-TAP): a multicenter survey to evaluate the percentages of dyslipidemic patients receiving lipid-lowering therapy and achieving low-density lipoprotein cholesterol goals. *Arch Intern Med* 2000; 160:459-67.

[22] McKee SA, Sane DC, Deliargyris EN. Aspirin resistance in cardiovascular disease: a review of prevalence, mechanisms, and clinical significance. *Thromb Haemost* 2002; 88:711-5.

[23] Poirier P, Eckel RH. Obesity and cardiovascular disease. *Curr Atheroscler Rep* 2002; 4:448-53.

[24] Flegal KM, Carroll MD, Ogden CL, Johnson CL. Prevalence and trends in obesity among US adults, 1999-2000. *JAMA* 2002; 288:1723-7.

[25] Mokdad AH, Ford ES, Bowman BA, Dietz WH, Vinicor F, et al. Prevalence of obesity, diabetes, and obesity-related health risk factors, 2001. *JAMA* 2003; 289:76-9.

[26] Dubbert PM, Carithers T, Sumner AE, Barbour KA, Clark BL, et al. Obesity, physical inactivity, and risk for cardiovascular disease. *Am J Med Sci* 2002; 324:116-26.

[27] Rozanski A, Blumenthal JA, Kaplan J. Impact of psychological factors on the pathogenesis of cardiovascular disease and implications for therapy. *Circulation* 1999; 99:2192-217.

[28] DeWood MA, Spores J, Notske R, Mouser LT, Burroughs R, et al. Prevalence of total coronary occlusion during the early hours of transmural myocardial infarction. *N Engl J Med* 1980; 303:897-902.

[29] Solomon HA, Edwards AL, Killip T. Prodromatan acute myocardial infarction. *Circulation* 1969; 40:463-71.

[30] Kannel WB, Schatzkin A. Sudden death: lessons from subsets in population studies. *J Am Coll Cardiol* 1985; 5:141B-149B.
[31] de Vreede-Swagemakers JJ, Gorgels AP, Dubois-Arbouw WI, van Ree JW, Daemen MJ, et al. Out-of-hospital cardiac arrest in the 1990's: a population-based study in the Maastricht area on incidence, characteristics and survival. *J Am Coll Cardiol* 1997; 30:1500-5.
[32] Ambrose JA, Tannenbaum MA, Alexopoulos D, Hjemdahl-Monsen CE, Leavy J, et al. Angiographic progression of coronary artery disease and the development of myocardial infarction. *J Am Coll Cardiol* 1988; 12:56-62.
[33] Herrick JB. Clinical features of sudden obstruction of the coronary arteries. *JAMA* 1912; 59:2015-2020.
[34] Willerson JT, Eidt JF, McNatt J, Yao SK, Golino P, et al. Role of thromboxane and serotonin as mediators in the development of spontaneous alterations in coronary blood flow and neointimal proliferation in canine models with chronic coronary artery stenoses and endothelial injury. *J Am Coll Cardiol* 1991; 17:101B-110B.
[35] Eidt JF, Allison P, Noble S, Ashton J, Golino P, et al. Thrombin is an important mediator of platelet aggregation in stenosed canine coronary arteries with endothelial injury. *J Clin Invest* 1989; 84:18-27.
[36] Ross R, Glomset JA. The pathogenesis of atherosclerosis (first of two parts). *N Engl J Med* 1976; 295:369-77.
[37] Ross R. Atherosclerosis--an inflammatory disease. *N Engl J Med* 1999; 340:115-26.
[38] Libby P, Geng YJ, Aikawa M, Schoenbeck U, Mach F, et al. Macrophages and atherosclerotic plaque stability. *Curr Opin Lipidol* 1996; 7:330-5.
[39] Rekhter MD. Collagen synthesis in atherosclerosis: too much and not enough. *Cardiovascular Research* 1999; 41:376-384.
[40] Shah PK. Mechanisms of plaque vulnerability and rupture. *J Am Coll Cardiol* 2003; 41:15S-22S.
[41] Friedman M, Van Den Bovenkamp GJ. The pathogenesis of a coronary thrombus. *Am J Pathol* 1966; 48:19-44.
[42] Farb A, Tang AL, Burke AP, Sessums L, Liang Y, Virmani R. Sudden coronary death. Frequency of active coronary lesions, inactive coronary lesions, and myocardial infarction. *Circulation* 1995; 92:1701-9.
[43] Falk E. Morphologic features of unstable atherothrombotic plaques underlying acute coronary syndromes. *Am J Cardiol* 1989; 63:114E-120E.
[44] Arbustini E, Dal Bello B, Morbini P, Burke AP, Bocciarelli M, et al. Plaque erosion is a major substrate for coronary thrombosis in acute myocardial infarction. *Heart* 1999; 82:269-72.
[45] Davies MJ, Thomas T. The pathological basis and microanatomy of occlusive thrombus formation in human coronary arteries. *Philos Trans R Soc Lond B Biol Sci* 1981; 294:225-9.
[46] Constantinides P. Plaque fissures in human coronary thrombosis. *J Atheroscler Res* 1966; 6:1-17.

[47] Virmani R, Kolodgie FD, Burke AP, Farb A, Schwartz SM. Lessons from sudden coronary death: a comprehensive morphological classification scheme for atherosclerotic lesions. *Arterioscler Thromb Vasc Biol* 2000; 20:1262-75.

[48] Hirsh PD, Campbell WB, Willerson JT, Hillis LD. Prostaglandins and ischemic heart disease. *Am J Med* 1981; 71:1009-26.

[49] Hirsh PD, Hillis LD, Campbell WB, Firth BG, Willerson JT. Release of prostaglandins and thromboxane into the coronary circulation in patients with ischemic heart disease. *N Engl J Med* 1981; 304:685-91.

[50] Fujise K, Stacy L, Beck P, Yeh ET, Chuang A, et al. Differential effects of endothelin receptor activation on cyclic flow variations in rat mesenteric arteries. *Circulation* 1997; 96:3641-6.

[51] Apprill P, Schmitz JM, Campbell WB, Tilton G, Ashton J, et al. Cyclic blood flow variations induced by platelet-activating factor in stenosed canine coronary arteries despite inhibition of thromboxane synthetase, serotonin receptors, and alpha-adrenergic receptors. *Circulation* 1985; 72:397-405.

[52] Guyton JR, Willerson JT. Peripheral venous platelet aggregates in patients with unstable angina pectoris and acute myocardial infarction. Angiology 1977; 28:695-701.

[53] Willerson JT. Conversion from chronic to acute coronary heart disease syndromes. Role of platelets and platelet products. *Tex Heart Inst J* 1995; 22:13-9.

[54] Willerson JT, Campbell WB, Winniford MD, Schmitz J, Apprill P, et al. Conversion from chronic to acute coronary artery disease: speculation regarding mechanisms. *Am J Cardiol* 1984; 54:1349-54.

[55] Little WC, Constantinescu M, Applegate RJ, Kutcher MA, Burrows MT, et al. Can coronary angiography predict the site of a subsequent myocardial infarction in patients with mild-to-moderate coronary artery disease? *Circulation* 1988; 78:1157-66.

[56] Hackett D, Davies G, Maseri A. Pre-existing coronary stenoses in patients with first myocardial infarction are not necessarily severe. *Eur Heart J* 1988; 9:1317-23.

[57] Lichtlen PR, Nikutta P, Jost S, Deckers J, Wiese B, Rafflenbeul W. Anatomical progression of coronary artery disease in humans as seen by prospective, repeated, quantitated coronary angiography. Relation to clinical events and risk factors. The INTACT Study Group. *Circulation* 1992; 86:828-38.

[58] Giroud D, Li JM, Urban P, Meier B, Rutishauer W. Relation of the site of acute myocardial infarction to the most severe coronary arterial stenosis at prior angiography. *Am J Cardiol* 1992; 69:729-32.

[59] Naqvi TZ, Hachamovitch R, Berman D, Buchbinder N, Kiat H, Shah PK. Does the presence and site of myocardial ischemia on perfusion scintigraphy predict the occurrence and site of future myocardial infarction in patients with stable coronary artery disease? *Am J Cardiol* 1997; 79:1521-4.

[60] Virchow R. Phlogose und thrombose in getissystem, gesanmelte unhandlungen zur wissensehaftlichen medlein. Frankfurt-am-Main, Germany: Meidinger Sohn, 1856:458.

[61] von Rokitansky C. *A manual of pathological anatomy*. Vol. Vol 4 [in orig lang]. London, UK: Sydenham Society, 1852:261.

[62] Herrick JB. Landmark article (JAMA 1912). Clinical features of sudden obstruction of the coronary arteries. *JAMA* 1983; 250:1757-65.
[63] Olcott CT. Rupture of a coronary artery, hemopericardium. Report of a case and review of the literature. *N Engl J Med* 1931; 204:760-763.
[64] Leary T. Pathology of coronary sclerosis. *Amer. Heart J.* 1934; 10:328-337.
[65] Wartman WB. Occlusion of coronary arteries by hemorrhage into their walls. *Am Heart J* 1938; 15:459-470.
[66] Blumgart HL, Schlesinger MJ, Davis D. Studies on the relation of the clinical manifestations of angina pectoris, coronary thrombosis, and myocardial infarction to the pathologic findings. *Am Heart J* 1940; 19:1-91.
[67] Chapman JM, Reeder LG, Massey FJ, Jr., Borun ER, Picken B, et al. Relationships of stress, tranquilizers, and serum cholesterol levels in a sample population under study for coronary heart disease. *Am J Epidemiol* 1966; 83:537-47.
[68] Farb A, Burke AP, Tang AL, Liang TY, Mannan P, et al. Coronary plaque erosion without rupture into a lipid core. A frequent cause of coronary thrombosis in sudden coronary death. *Circulation* 1996; 93:1354-63.
[69] Burke AP, Farb A, Malcom GT, Liang Y, Smialek JE, Virmani R. Plaque rupture and sudden death related to exertion in men with coronary artery disease. *JAMA* 1999; 281:921-6.
[70] Kolodgie FD, Burke AP, Farb A, Gold HK, Yuan J, et al. The thin-cap fibroatheroma: a type of vulnerable plaque: the major precursor lesion to acute coronary syndromes. *Curr Opin Cardiol* 2001; 16:285-92.
[71] Pasterkamp G, Schoneveld AH, van der Wal AC, Hijnen DJ, van Wolveren WJ, et al. Inflammation of the atherosclerotic cap and shoulder of the plaque is a common and locally observed feature in unruptured plaques of femoral and coronary arteries. *Arterioscler Thromb Vasc Biol* 1999; 19:54-8.
[72] Burleigh MC, Briggs AD, Lendon CL, Davies MJ, Born GV, Richardson PD. Collagen types I and III, collagen content, GAGs and mechanical strength of human atherosclerotic plaque caps: span-wise variations. *Atherosclerosis* 1992; 96:71-81.
[73] Burke AP, Kolodgie FD, Farb A, Weber DK, Malcom GT, et al. Healed plaque ruptures and sudden coronary death : Evidence that subclinical rupture has a role in plaque progression. *Circulation* 2001; 103:934-940.
[74] Uchida Y, Nakamura F, Tomaru T, Morita T, Oshima T, et al. Prediction of acute coronary syndromes by percutaneous coronary angioscopy in patients with stable angina. *Am Heart J* 1995; 130:195-203.
[75] Nobuyoshi M, Tanaka M, Nosaka H, Kimura T, Yokoi H, et al. Progression of coronary atherosclerosis: is coronary spasm related to progression? *J Am Coll Cardiol* 1991; 18:904-10.
[76] Haft JI, al-Zarka AM. The origin and fate of complex coronary lesions. *Am Heart J* 1991; 121:1050-61.
[77] Kimbiris D, Lavine P, Van Den Broek H, Najmi M, Likoff W. Devolutionary pattern of coronary atherosclerosis in patients with angina pectoris. Coronary arteriographic studies. *Am J Cardiol* 1974; 33:7-11.

[78] Mocetti T, Lichtlen P, Schonbeck M, Steinbrunn W. *Progression of coronary artery disease based on cine angiographic data.* In: Lichtlen PR, ed. Coronary Angiography and Angina Pectoris (Symposium of the European Society of Cardiology). Stuttgart: Georg Thieme, 1976:88-97.

[79] McLaughlin PR, Berman ND, Morton BC, Schwartz L, Morch JE. Long-term angiographic assessment of the influence of coronary risk factors on native coronary circulation and saphenous vein aortocoronary grafts. *Am Heart J* 1977; 93:327-33.

[80] Marchandise B, Bourassa MG, Chaitman BR, Lesperance J. Angiographic evaluation of the natural history of normal coronary arteries and mild coronary atherosclerosis. *Am J Cardiol* 1978; 41:216-20.

[81] Shub C, Vlietstra RE, Smith HC, Fulton RE, Elveback LR. The unpredictable progression of symptomatic coronary artery disease: a serial clinical-angiographic analysis. *Mayo Clin Proc* 1981; 56:155-60.

[82] Yokoya K, Takatsu H, Suzuki T, Hosokawa H, Ojio S, et al. Process of progression of coronary artery lesions from mild or moderate stenosis to moderate or severe stenosis : A study based on four serial coronary arteriograms per year. *Circulation* 1999; 100:903-909.

[83] Veen G, Meyer A, Verheugt FW, Werter CJ, de Swart H, et al. Culprit lesion morphology and stenosis severity in the prediction of reocclusion after coronary thrombolysis: angiographic results of the APRICOT study. Antithrombotics in the Prevention of Reocclusion in Coronary Thrombolysis. *J Am Coll Cardiol* 1993; 22:1755-62.

[84] Chen L, Chester MR, Redwood S, Huang J, Leatham E, Kaski JC. Angiographic stenosis progression and coronary events in patients with 'stabilized' unstable angina. *Circulation* 1995; 91:2319-24.

[85] Brown BG, Zhao XQ, Sacco DE, Albers JJ. Atherosclerosis regression, plaque disruption, and cardiovascular events: a rationale for lipid lowering in coronary artery disease. *Annu Rev Med* 1993; 44:365-76.

[86] Libby P, Aikawa M. New insights into plaque stabilisation by lipid lowering. *Drugs* 1998; 56 Suppl 1:9-13; discussion 33.

[87] Moise A, Lesperance J, Theroux P, Taeymans Y, Goulet C, Bourassa MG. Clinical and angiographic predictors of new total coronary occlusion in coronary artery disease: analysis of 313 nonoperated patients. *Am J Cardiol* 1984; 54:1176-81.

[88] Singh RN. Progression of coronary atherosclerosis. Clues to pathogenesis from serial coronary arteriography. *Br Heart J* 1984; 52:451-61.

[89] Brown BG, Gallery CA, Badger RS, Kennedy JW, Mathey D, et al. Incomplete lysis of thrombus in the moderate underlying atherosclerotic lesion during intracoronary infusion of streptokinase for acute myocardial infarction: quantitative angiographic observations. *Circulation* 1986; 73:653-61.

[90] Alderman EL, Corley SD, Fisher LD, Chaitman BR, Faxon DP, et al. Five-year angiographic follow-up of factors associated with progression of coronary artery disease in the Coronary Artery Surgery Study (CASS). CASS Participating Investigators and Staff. *J Am Coll Cardiol* 1993; 22:1141-54.

[91] Freeman MR, Williams AE, Chisholm RJ, Armstrong PW. Intracoronary thrombus and complex morphology in unstable angina. Relation to timing of angiography and in-hospital cardiac events. *Circulation* 1989; 80:17-23.
[92] Davies SW, Marchant B, Lyons JP, Timmis AD, Rothman MT, et al. Irregular coronary lesion morphology after thrombolysis predicts early clinical instability. *J Am Coll Cardiol* 1991; 18:669-74.
[93] Davies MJ. Stability and instability: two faces of coronary atherosclerosis. The Paul Dudley White Lecture 1995. *Circulation* 1996; 94:2013-20.
[94] Joseph A, Talley JD, Shih A, Crum T, Vogel R, Kupersmith J. Clinical and angiographic variables affecting the progression of coronary artery disease as determined by quantitative angiography. *Int J Card Imaging* 1994; 10:217-25.
[95] Ellis S, Alderman EL, Cain K, Wright A, Bourassa M, Fisher L. Morphology of left anterior descending coronary territory lesions as a predictor of anterior myocardial infarction: a CASS Registry Study. *J Am Coll Cardiol* 1989; 13:1481-91.
[96] Guazzi MD, Bussotti M, Grancini L, De Cesare N, Guazzi M, et al. Evidence of multifocal activity of coronary disease in patients with acute myocardial infarction. *Circulation* 1997; 96:1145-51.
[97] Ambrose JA. Prognostic implications of lesion irregularity on coronary angiography. *J Am Coll Cardiol* 1991; 18:675-6.
[98] Ozaki Y, Keane D, Serruys PW. Progression and regression of coronary stenosis in the long-term follow-up of vasospastic angina. *Circulation* 1995; 92:2446-56.
[99] Kaski JC, Chester MR, Chen L, Katritsis D. Rapid angiographic progression of coronary artery disease in patients with angina pectoris. The role of complex stenosis morphology. *Circulation* 1995; 92:2058-65.
[100] Malek AM, Alper SL, Izumo S. Hemodynamic shear stress and its role in atherosclerosis. *JAMA* 1999; 282:2035-42.
[101] Gibson CM, Diaz L, Kandarpa K, Sacks FM, Pasternak RC, et al. Relation of vessel wall shear stress to atherosclerosis progression in human coronary arteries. *Arterioscler Thromb* 1993; 13:310-5.
[102] Gertz SD, Roberts WC. Hemodynamic shear force in rupture of coronary arterial atherosclerotic plaques. *Am J Cardiol* 1990; 66:1368-72.
[103] Traub O, Berk BC. Laminar shear stress: mechanisms by which endothelial cells transduce an atheroprotective force. *Arterioscler Thromb Vasc Biol* 1998; 18:677-85.
[104] Chappell DC, Varner SE, Nerem RM, Medford RM, Alexander RW. Oscillatory shear stress stimulates adhesion molecule expression in cultured human endothelium. *Circ Res* 1998; 82:532-9.
[105] Zarins CK, Bomberger RA, Glagov S. Local effects of stenoses: increased flow velocity inhibits atherogenesis. *Circulation* 1981; 64:II221-7.
[106] Schwartz CJ, Mitchell JRA. Observations on localization of arterial plaques. *Circ Res* 1962; 11:63-73.
[107] Badimon L, Badimon JJ, Galvez A, Chesebro JH, Fuster V. Influence of arterial damage and wall shear rate on platelet deposition. Ex vivo study in a swine model. *Arteriosclerosis* 1986; 6:312-20.

[108] Friedman MH, Bargeron CB, Deters OJ, Hutchins GM, Mark FF. Correlation between wall shear and intimal thickness at a coronary artery branch. *Atherosclerosis* 1987; 68:27-33.

[109] Casscells W, Hassan K, Vasegi MF, Siadaty MS, Naghavi M, et al. Plaque blush, branch location, and calcification are angiographic predictors of progression of mild to moderate coronary stenoses. *Am Heart J* 2003; 145:813-20.

[110] Moulton KS, Heller E, Konerding MA, Flynn E, Palinski W, Folkman J. Angiogenesis inhibitors endostatin or TNP-470 reduce intimal neovascularization and plaque growth in Apolipoprotein E–deficient mice. *Circulation* 1999; 99:1726-1732.

[111] Alpern-Elran H, Morog N, Robert F, Hoover G, Kalant N, Brem S. Angiogenic activity of the atherosclerotic carotid artery plaque. *J Neurosurg* 1989; 70:942-5.

[112] Depre C, Havaux X, Wijns W. Neovascularization in human coronary atherosclerotic lesions. *Cathet Cardiovasc Diagn* 1996; 39:215-20.

[113] O'Brien ER, Garvin MR, Dev R, Stewart DK, Hinohara T, et al. Angiogenesis in human coronary atherosclerotic plaques. *Am J Pathol* 1994; 145:883-94.

[114] Mizuno K, Miyamoto A, Satomura K, Kurita A, Arai T, et al. Angioscopic coronary macromorphology in patients with acute coronary disorders. *Lancet* 1991; 337:809-12.

[115] Thieme T, Wernecke KD, Meyer R, Brandenstein E, Habedank D, et al. Angioscopic evaluation of atherosclerotic plaques: validation by histomorphologic analysis and association with stable and unstable coronary syndromes. *J Am Coll Cardiol* 1996; 28:1-6.

Sherman CT, Litvack F, Grundfest W, Lee M, Hickey A, et al. Coronary angioscopy in patients with unstable angina pectoris. *N Engl J Med* 1986; 315:913-9.

[116] Asakura M, Ueda Y, Yamaguchi O, Adachi T, Hirayama A, et al. Extensive development of vulnerable plaques as a pan-coronary process in patients with myocardial infarction: an angioscopic study. *J Am Coll Cardiol* 2001; 37:1284-8.

[117] Waxman S, Sassower MA, Mittleman MA, Zarich S, Miyamoto A, et al. Angioscopic predictors of early adverse outcome after coronary angioplasty in patients with unstable angina and non-Q-wave myocardial infarction. *Circulation* 1996; 93:2106-13.

[118] de Feyter PJ, Ozaki Y, Baptista J, Escaned J, Di Mario C, et al. Ischemia-related lesion characteristics in patients with stable or unstable angina. A study with intracoronary angioscopy and ultrasound. *Circulation* 1995; 92:1408-13.

[119] Van Belle E, Lablanche JM, Bauters C, Renaud N, McFadden EP, Bertrand ME. Coronary angioscopic findings in the infarct-related vessel within 1 month of acute myocardial infarction: natural history and the effect of thrombolysis. *Circulation* 1998; 97:26-33.

[120] Casscells W, Hathorn B, David M, Krabach T, Vaughn WK, et al. Thermal detection of cellular infiltrates in living atherosclerotic plaques: possible implications for plaque rupture and thrombosis. *Lancet* 1996; 347:1447-51.

[121] Madjid M, Naghavi N, Willerson JT, Casscells W. *Thermography: A novel approach for identification of plaques at risk of rupture and/or thrombosis*. In: Fuster V, ed. Assessing and Modifying the Vulnerable Atherosclerotic Plaque. Armonk, NY: Futura Publishing Company, Inc., 2002:107-127.

[122] Stefanadis C, Diamantopoulos L, Vlachopoulos C, Tsiamis E, Dernellis J, et al. Thermal heterogeneity within human atherosclerotic coronary arteries detected in vivo: A new method of detection by application of a special thermography catheter. *Circulation* 1999; 99:1965-71.

[123] Stefanadis C, Diamantopoulos L, Dernellis J, Economou E, Tsiamis E, et al. Heat production of atherosclerotic plaques and inflammation assessed by the acute phase proteins in acute coronary syndromes. *J Mol Cell Cardiol* 2000; 32:43-52.

[124] Stefanadis C, Toutouzas K, Tsiamis E, Stratos C, Vavuranakis M, et al. Increased local temperature in human coronary atherosclerotic plaques: an independent predictor of clinical outcome in patients undergoing a percutaneous coronary intervention. *J Am Coll Cardiol* 2001; 37:1277-83.

[125] Stefanadis C, Toutouzas K, Vavuranakis M, Tsiamis E, Tousoulis D, et al. Statin treatment is associated with reduced thermal heterogeneity in human atherosclerotic plaques. *Eur Heart J* 2002; 23:1664-9.

[126] Verheye S, Van Langenhove G, Diamantopoulos L, Serruys PW, Vermeersch P. Temperature heterogeneity is nearly absent in angiographically normal or mild atherosclerotic coronary segments: Interim results from a safety study (abstract). *Am J Cardiol* 2002; 90:24H.

[127] Webster M, Stewart J, Ruygrok P, Ormiston J, Scott D, et al. Intracoronary thermogrophy with a multiple thermocouple catheter: Initial human experience (abstract). *Am J Cardiol* 2002; 90:24H.

[128] Toutouzas MK, Stefanadis CM, Vavuranakis MM, Tsiamis ME, Tsioufis MC, et al. Arterial remodeling in acute coronary syndromes: correlation of IVUS characteristics with temperature of the culprit lesion. *Circulation* 2000; 102:II-707.

[129] Toutouzas K, Stefanadis C, Tsiamis E, Vavuranakis M, Tsioufis C, et al. The temperature of atherosclerotic plaques is correlated with matrix metalloproteinases concentration in patients with acute coronary syndromes. *J Am Coll Cardiol* 2001; 37:356A.

[130] Verheye S, De Meyer GRY, Van Langenhove G, Knaapen MWM, Kockx MM. In vivo temperature heterogeneity of atherosclerotic plaques Is determined by plaque composition. *Circulation* 2002; 105:1596-1601.

[131] Rioufol G, Finet G, Ginon I, Andre-Fouet X, Rossi R, et al. Multiple atherosclerotic plaque rupture in acute coronary syndrome: a three-vessel intravascular ultrasound study. *Circulation* 2002; 106:804-8.

[132] Ge J, Chirillo F, Schwedtmann J, Gorge G, Haude M, et al. Screening of ruptured plaques in patients with coronary artery disease by intravascular ultrasound. *Heart* 1999; 81:621-7.

[133] Schaar JA, de Korte CL, Mastik F, Baldewsing R, Regar E, et al. Intravascular palpography for high-risk vulnerable plaque assessment. *Herz* 2003; 28:488-95.

[134] Schaar JA, De Korte CL, Mastik F, Strijder C, Pasterkamp G, et al. Characterizing vulnerable plaque features with intravascular elastography. *Circulation* 2003; 108:2636-41.

[135] Brezinski M. Characterizing arterial plaque with optical coherence tomography. *Curr Opin Cardiol* 2002; 17:648-655.

[136] Jang IK, Bouma BE, Kang DH, Park SJ, Park SW, et al. Visualization of coronary atherosclerotic plaques in patients using optical coherence tomography: comparison with intravascular ultrasound. *J Am Coll Cardiol* 2002; 39:604-9.

[137] Raggi P. Role of coronary calcium screening in preventive cardiology. *Prev Cardiol* 2003; 6:214-7.

[138] Shaw LJ, Raggi P, Schisterman E, Berman DS, Callister TQ. Prognostic value of cardiac risk factors and coronary artery calcium screening for all-cause mortality. *Radiology* 2003; 228:826-33.

[139] Litovsky SH, Min SH, Naghavi M, Payvar S, Casscells SW. Macrophages colocalize with neovascularization and calcification in carotid endarterectomy specimens: Implications for plaque destabilization (abstract). *Am J Cardiol* 2002; 90:113H.

[140] Fayad ZA, Choudhury RP, Fuster V. Magnetic resonance imaging of coronary atherosclerosis. *Curr Atheroscler Rep* 2003; 5:411-7.

[141] Flacke S, Fischer S, Scott MJ, Fuhrhop RJ, Allen JS, et al. Novel MRI contrast agent for molecular imaging of fibrin: implications for detecting vulnerable plaques. *Circulation* 2001; 104:1280-5.

[142] Fayad ZA, Fuster V. The human high-risk plaque and its detection by magnetic resonance imaging. *Am J Cardiol* 2001; 88:42E-45E.

[143] Yuan C, Mitsumori LM, Beach KW, Maravilla KR. Carotid atherosclerotic plaque: noninvasive MR characterization and identification of vulnerable lesions. *Radiology* 2001; 221:285-99.

[144] Ruehm SG, Corot C, Vogt P, Kolb S, Debatin JF. Magnetic resonance imaging of atherosclerotic plaque with ultrasmall superparamagnetic particles of iron oxide in hyperlipidemic rabbits. *Circulation* 2001; 103:415-422.

[145] Major outcomes in high-risk hypertensive patients randomized to angiotensin-converting enzyme inhibitor or calcium channel blocker vs diuretic: The Antihypertensive and Lipid-Lowering Treatment to Prevent Heart Attack Trial (ALLHAT). *JAMA* 2002; 288:2981-97.

[146] The sixth report of the Joint National Committee on prevention, detection, evaluation, and treatment of high blood pressure. *Arch Intern Med* 1997; 157:2413-46.

[147] Messerli FH. Hypertension and sudden cardiac death. *Am J Hypertens* 1999; 12:181S-188S.

[148] Kuller LH, Ockene JK, Meilahn E, Wentworth DN, Svendsen KH, Neaton JD. Cigarette smoking and mortality. MRFIT Research Group. *Prev Med* 1991; 20:638-54.

[149] Ambrose JA, Tannenbaum MA, Alexopoulos D, Hjemdahl-Monsen CE, Leavy J, et al. Angiographic progression of coronary artery disease and the development of myocardial infarction. *J Am Coll Cardiol* 1988; 12:56-62.

Acknowledgements

This work is supported in part by the DREAMS program of the Department of Defense (Grant #DAMD 17-01-2-0047 to Dr. S. Ward Casscells).

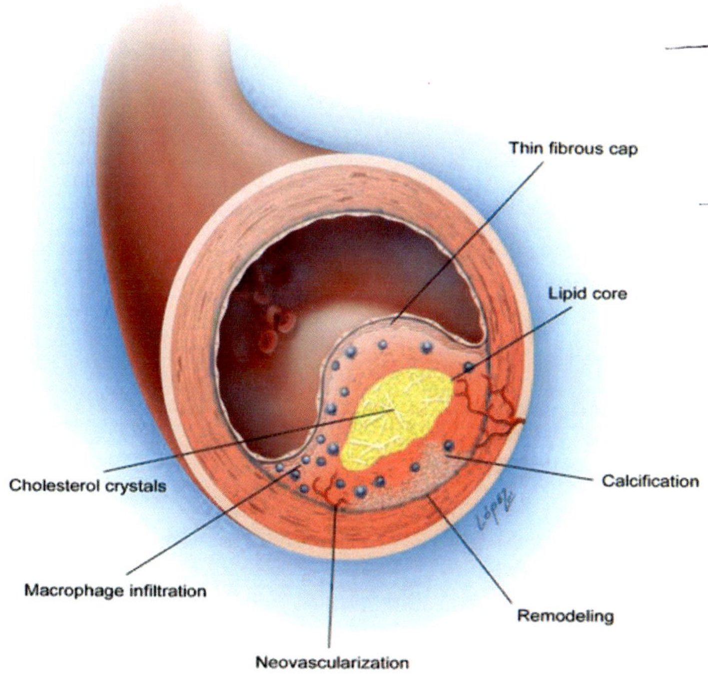

Figure 1. Histopathological features of vulnerable atherosclerotic plaques include a thin fibrous cap, a large lipid core, mild to moderate deep calcification, outward remodeling, neovascularization, and infiltration of inflammatory cells, especially at the shoulder region.

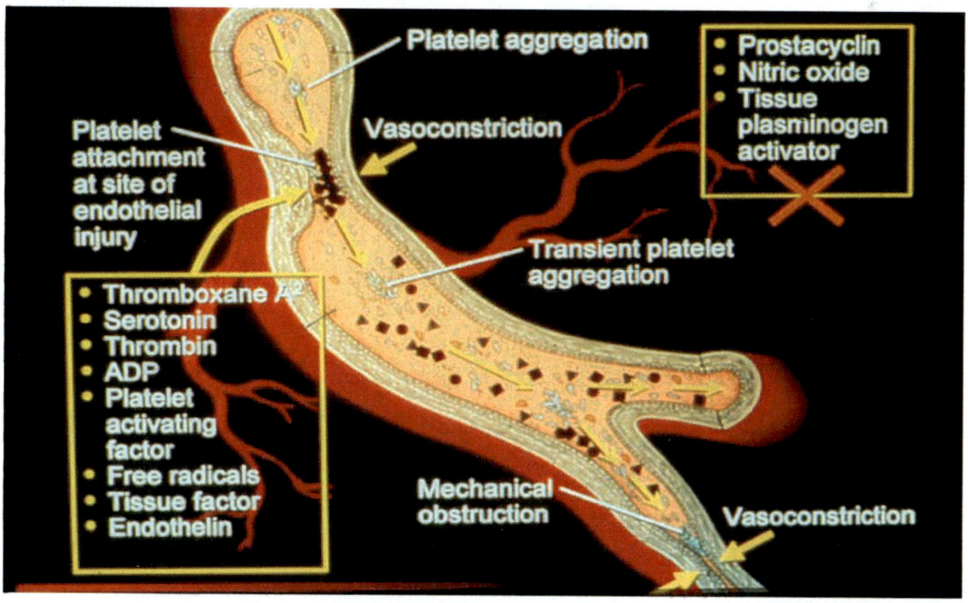

Figure 2. Arterial injury, platelet aggregation, transient thrombosis and vasoconstriction lead to unstable angina and myocardial infarction. (Adapted from Willerson JT, Cohn JN. Cardiovascular Medicine. Philadelphia: Churchill Livingstone, 2000).

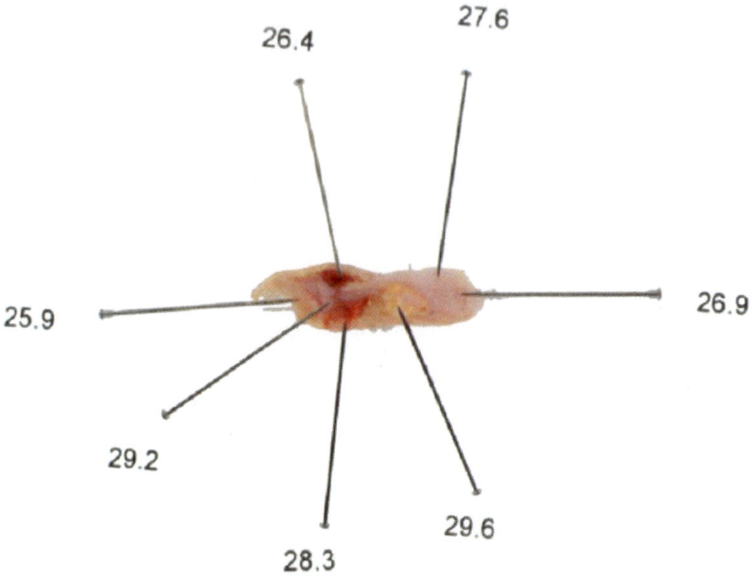

Figure 3. Endarterectomized carotid plaques show temperature heterogeneity. (Reprinted with permission from Madjid et al. in Fuster V. (ed). Assessing and modifying the vulnerable atherosclerotic plaque. Armonk, NY: Futura Publishing Company, Inc. 2002).

In: Current Topics in Atherosclerosis Research
Editor: Yong J. Geng, pp. 23-47

ISBN 1-59454-428-X

Chapter II

Vascular Cell Apoptosis in Atherosclerotic Plaque

Yong-Jian Geng*

The Center for Cardiovascular Biology and Atherosclerosis Research, Department of Internal Medicine, University of Texas Health Science Center at Houston, Houston, TX

Abstract

During the development of atherosclerosis, the arterial tissue undergoes contant remodeling and changes in cellularity. Increasing evidence from pathological studies indicates different roles that apoptosis, a form of programmed cell death, plays in different phases of atherosclerosis. Physiologically, the arterial wall removes unwanted, aging or injured cells by apoptosis. In early stages of atherosclerosis, apoptosis reduces accumulation of cellular components in the intima, thus preventing intimal thickness. In advanced plaques, to a certain degree, apoptosis eliminates inflammatory cells and reduces foam cell formation. However, accelerated apoptosis delete healthy vascular cells and reduce the capacity of vascular tissue repair, and even trigger plaque rupture, an event leading to acute vascular syndromes. At cellular levels, both vascular cells and non-vascular cells may undergo apoptosis, albeit under different mechanisms. Interactions between vascular cells and inflammatory cells, mainly macrophages and lymphocytes, contribute to vascular cell death. There are multiple molecular pathways by which extracellular and intracellular molecules induce vascular cell apoptosis. Oxidized lipoproteins and their lipid components are the primary pro-apoptotic substances that exist abundantly in atherosclerotic lesions. Proinflammatory cytokines produced by activated macrophages and T lymphocytes are also pro-apoptotic. Oxidized lipids and cytotoxic cytokines may synergize to trigger apoptosis of smooth muscle cells. Two cell

* Correspondence concerning this article should be addressed to Dr. Yong-Jian Geng, the Center for Cardiovascular Biology and Atherosclerosis Research, Division of Cardiology, Department of Internal Medeicine, University of Texas Health Science Center at Houston, Houston, TX77030. Email: yong-jian.geng@uth.tmc.edu

death signaling pathways have been documented in vascular cells; 1) the non-receptor mediated, mitochondria-associated caspase activation and 2) the death receptor-mediated, autoproteolytic caspase activation. There is also interplay between internal genes and a variety of anti- and pro-apoptotic factors in atherosclerotic arteries. Imbalance between apoptosis and procreation may ultimately alter the cellularity of the arterial wall. Clarification of these pathways may aid development of novel therapeutic strategies to treat atherosclerosis and its complications, including the acute coronary syndromes.

Color graphics are presented at the end of the chapter.

Keywords: Atherosclerosis; Apoptosis; Smooth muscle cells; Caspase; Inflammation.

INTRODUCTION

Together with lipid deposition and connective tissue formation, increased accumulation of cellular components promotes thickness of the intima of arteries, a key pathological alteration during the development of atherosclerotic plaques. However, the increased cell mass in the intima does not reflect the rates of cell growth and death. Over the long-lasting process of atherogenesis often for several decades, many plaque cells may undergo apoptosis, a form of programmed cell death. [1] Indeed, cells may die in various ways, apoptotic or non-apoptotic (Table 1). Cell death may occur in a disorganized and chaotic energy-independent manner, associated with swelling, in response to lethal injury known as necrosis or, more properly, oncosis. [2] In contrast, cell death by apoptosis occurs in a coordinated and highly regulated fashion that involves shrinkage, not swelling. Apoptosis requires expression of certain groups of genes critical for cellular signal transduction and metabolism. This process provides a major mechanism by which tissues remove unwanted, aged, or damaged cells. Because of its ordered sequence of events, investigators often refer to apoptosis as *Programmed Cell Death*. Different cell types undergoing apoptosis in tissues and cultures share very similar morphologic features, including chromatin compaction and margination, nuclear condensation and fragmentation, and cell body shrinkage and blebbing (Table 1). These characteristic morphological alterations in apoptotic cells, which differ from those seen in necrotic cell death, reflect the self-directed catabolism of cytoskeleton and other intracellular molecules. Complex interactions between extracellular microenvironmental factors and intrinsic gene products occur before apoptosis begins. Once activated, this process can progress in the absence of extracellular insults. This suicidal feature of apoptosis applies to embryonic development and morphogenesis as well as adult tissue turnover. Apoptotic cells or bodies usually retain an intact cellular membrane and undergo prompt removal by tissue macrophages or adjacent cells, thus avoiding damage to neighboring tissue and triggering inflammation. Various methodologies can evaluate apoptosis in vivo and in vitro, including analysis of morphology, DNA fragmentation (e.g., *in situ* DNA terminase-mediated dUTP nick 3'end labeling of DNA fragments or TUNEL, and agarose gel electrophoresis), and immunolocalization of active forms of effector proteins. Many of these methods have significant limitations. For example, avoidance of artifacts with the TUNEL method requires special care. [3] However, because no single validated marker for apoptosis exists, its assessment ideally uses a combination of molecular and morphologic methods.

In 1995, we and others [4-6] provided morphological and biochemical evidence for apoptotic cell death in human advanced atherosclerotic plaques. In addition, we colocalized the prototypical caspase, caspase-1 or interleukin-1β converting enzyme, to sites of apoptosis in human atheroma. These early studies demonstrated the occurrence of apoptosis in both macrophages and SMC, two cell types that replicate prominently during atherogenesis. We further showed that the Fas/TNF caspase death-signaling pathway operates in human atherosclerotic lesions and may participate in vascular cell death during progression of atherosclerosis. [7,8] Experimental atheroma in rabbits fed a high cholesterol diet also demonstrated apoptosis.[9] Since then, numerous investigations have documented vascular cell apoptosis during the development of atherosclerosis and its complications (e.g., the acute coronary syndromes).

Table 1. Differences in morphology and biochemistry between apoptosis and oncosis (necrosis)

	Apoptosis	Oncosis
Triggers	External/Internal	External
Dying cells	Individual	Group
Death process	Programmed	Accidental
Cell body	Shrinking	Swelling
Plasma membrane	Intact	Broken
Lysosome	Intact	Leaking
Cytoskeleton	Collapse before death	Collapse after death
Mitochondria	Intact with Cyt-c release and ATP synthesis	Broken without ATP synthesis
Nucleus	Shrinking and fragmented	Enlarged and broken
Chromatin	Condensation	Clumping
DNA	Internucleosomal fragmentation	Randomized fragmentation
Caspases	Early activation	Uncertain
Inflammation	Rare	Common

This chapter aims to delineate the relationship of cell proliferation with atherogenesis and the molecular mechanisms that regulate apoptotic vascular cell death during the progression or regression of atheroma and the development of the acute coronary syndromes.

The Proliferation Paradox in Atherogenesis

Formation of the intimal macrophage-rich fatty streak, the precursor of atherosclerotic lesions, appears ubiquitous in humans. However, not all fatty streaks evolve into advanced lesions, i.e., fibrous plaques or atheroma. Thus, the mere accumulation of lipid-laden macrophages within the arterial intima does not ineluctably lead to formation of complicated atherosclerotic plaques. Depending upon the balance between pro-atherogenic and anti-atherogenic factors, some fatty streaks progress into atheroma and others may regress. The progression of fatty streaks to more complex lesions requires not only inflammatory cell infiltration but also the participation of SMC, a principal source of the extracellular matrix that ultimately often comprises the majority of the advanced atheroma's volume.

For decades, much of the research in the cell biology of atherosclerosis have centered on smooth muscle replication. Platelet-derived growth factor (PDGF) received much attention as a potential mitogenic stimulus during atheroma formation. Yet, PDGF *in vivo* appears more important as a chemoattractant for SMC than as a mitogen. [10] Moreover, the proliferation of SMC in human atherosclerotic lesions appears indolent, although bursts of SMC replication may indeed occur during atherogenesis. For example, episodes of localized plaque disruption with mural thrombosis or microvascular rupture within a plaque could stimulate a round of SMC proliferation due to thrombin or PDGF stimulation [11,12]. Transforming growth factor-β (TGFβ) released from platelet granules might, however, mitigate this mitogenesis due to its cytostatic action [13]. Interferon-γ (IFNγ) produced by T lymphocytes and other cells within plaques can also retard SMC proliferation by a cytostatic effect [14]. Macrophages proliferate within atheroma as well, no doubt due in part to the action of mitogens and co-mitogens such as monocyte-colony stimulating factor (M-CSF) or granulocyte-monocyte-colony stimulating factor (GM-CSF). Despite the operation of proliferation and cytostatic stimuli in atheroma, a full understanding of the regulation of plaque cellularity requires consideration of cell death, the topic of the balance of this essay.

Apoptosis in the Regulation of Cellularity of Atherosclerotic Arteries

Atherosclerotic lesions develop in the tunica intima of the arteries where accumulation of cellular components, lipids, and extracellular matrix yields a fibrofatty plaque that focally thickens the artery wall and can ultimately narrow the lumen. By counterbalancing proliferation, apoptosis may limit cell build-up in the intimal compartment. Elimination of lipid-laden foam cells may lead to the regression of atherosclerosis.

In contrast, attenuation of apoptosis may increase the tissue cellularity and promote intimal hyperplasia. Recent studies suggest the possibility that an anti-apoptotic mechanism may favor foam cell accumulation in atherosclerotic lesions. [15] Despite its harsh environment, many lipid-laden foam macrophages reside in the plaque's lipid core. Expression of anti-apoptotic genes may partially explain the apparent resistance of these foam cells to apoptosis. We have recently found that engagement of the class A or B scavenger receptor responsible for uptake of chemically modified lipoproteins can protect cultured macrophages from apoptosis induced by oxysterols and oxidized low-density lipoprotein (oxLDL). [16] The mechanism by which this scavenger receptor inhibits apoptosis in macrophages remains uncertain. Some evidence implies that the scavenger receptor-associated resistance of foam cells to apoptosis involves altered signal transduction, since expression of this receptor inhibits apoptosis induced by sodium fluoride, a global activator of GTP-binding proteins [17].

Apoptosis can occur during different stages of the development and evolution of advanced atherosclerotic lesions or atheroma [18]. In addition to lipids and connective tissue, the center of the typical atherosclerotic plaque contains many dead cells or cell debris, hence the term 'necrotic' or lipid core. Apoptosis causes cell loss as atherosclerosis progresses, often yielding a late or mature lesion containing a dense extracellular matrix with a relatively sparse cell population. Analysis of cell death by *in situ* end-labeling of DNA fragments (TUNEL technique) and by morphological observation indicates that many cells in the atheromatous lesions bear the markers of apoptosis even though necrotic cell death may also occur in the lipid core area of atherosclerotic lesions. [6] Thus, apoptosis may contribute to the formation of two major pathological changes characteristic of advanced atherosclerotic plaques, the 'necrotic lipid core' and the hypocellular fibrotic lesion.

Many laboratories reported a high percentage of apoptotic cells in advanced, progressive atherosclerotic plaques. Because the tissue volume should decrease when the levels of apoptosis exceed that of proliferation, this finding poses a paradox. However, the presence of markers of apoptosis may not always link with reduction of tissue volume. This situation could occur if the markers employed to assess apoptosis did not reflect an increase in the instantaneous rates of cell death. Indeed, accumulation of apoptotic cells in the plaques suggests that the system for scavenging the dead cells operates poorly in atherosclerosis. Some apoptotic cells or bodies in the plaques may remain 'mummified' rather than being removed by phagocytosis. [6] The following mechanisms might lead to retention of apoptotic cells or bodies in atherosclerotic lesions: (1) intracellular accumulation of lipids may attenuate the ability of macrophages and SMC to engulf and digest apoptotic cells; (2) phagocytosis may decrease due to increased apoptosis of macrophages in the lesions; (3) cross-linking of macromolecules such as proteins, nucleic acid, and carbohydrates may stabilize apoptotic cells in the tissues [19]; and (4) increased amounts of chemically modified lipoproteins and other ligands for scavenger receptors may competitively block the receptor-mediated phagocytosis of apoptotic cells by macrophages. In addition, recent studies have provided evidence that increased calcification and fibrosis may occur in atherosclerotic lesions with that contain apoptotic cells or bodies.

Apoptosis and the Stability of Atherosclerotic Plaques

Plaque disruption frequently causes the thrombotic complications of atherosclerosis that underlie unstable angina pectoris, myocardial infarction, and other acute syndromes. [20-22] Vascular SMC can synthesize a variety of extracellular matrix macromolecules that stabilize the plaques. Inflammatory cell accumulation characterizes disrupted plaques. [23,24] Production of apoptosis-promoting mediators by activated inflammatory or immune cells may lead to death of vascular SMC, which may in turn weaken and destabilize the plaques. Indeed, in 1995 we dubbed SMC 'the guardians of the integrity of the plaque's fibrous cap', and we originally proposed a role for SMC drop-out due to apoptosis in thinning of the fibrous cap.[25]

Either apoptotic EC [26] or SMC [27] can promote coagulation. Rapid exposure of membrane phosphatidylserine and loss of the anticoagulant membrane components in apoptotic EC can occur, which may promote a pro-coagulant environment. Apoptotic vascular SMC acquire thrombin-generating capacity due to exposure of phosphatidylserine. Apoptotic cells within atherosclerotic plaques may thus allow local thrombin activation, thereby contributing to disease progression. [27] Increased tissue factor on the surface of apoptotic cells may also contribute to the procoagulant activities [28]. These findings illustrate how apoptotic cells or bodies, if not promptly removed, may become thrombogenic or pro-inflammatory.

Although apoptosis usually occurs more frequently in the intimal cells, under certain pathological conditions this type of cell death may attack medial SMC. In association with p53 expression, the medial SMC of arteries with aneurysms exhibit considerable levels of apoptosis [29]. Macrophages and T lymphocytes infiltrate the arterial wall in atherosclerotic aortic aneurysms and produce death-promoting proteins (perforin, Fas, and FasL). [30] Thus, accelerated apoptosis of medial SMC represents a cellular mechanism responsible for the development of aortic aneurysms.

Pro-Apoptotic Factors Operating During Atherogenesis

Vascular SMC and EC encounter a broad variety of biologically active environmental factors such as mechanical force [31-35], oxidative stress [36], radiation [37-41], reactive oxygen or nitrogen species [42-45], lipids (cholesterol and its oxides) [16,41,46-48], viral [49-51] and bacterial products [52] as well as inflammatory cytokines [7,53,54] produced by activated immune cells. Many of these extracellular environmental and immunological factors can induce apoptosis in vascular cells (Table 2).

Atherosclerotic lesions contain chemically modified lipoproteins, in particular oxidized low-density lipoprotein (oxLDL), a putative instigator of atherosclerosis inducing vascular cell apoptosis [48]. Intrinsically, cholesterol and its esters have little pro-apoptotic action, but they become cytotoxic after oxidation. Some oxysterols [47] in oxLDL particles may contribute to the pro-apoptotic action of oxLDL. High levels of cholesterol oxides in the cell membrane can trigger foam cell death by apoptosis [55]. Oxysterol-mediated apoptosis may foster formation of a necrotic lipid core, a region with relatively high concentrations of oxysterols. [56] Mechanisms by which oxLDL and oxysterols may trigger apoptosis remain incompletely understood. Recent studies suggest that activation of caspases [46] and sphingomyelinase [57], attenuation of Bcl2 [46], and suppression of the nuclear transcription factor NF-κB [58] may contribute to oxLDL-induced apoptosis.

Beyond lipid accumulation, atherogenesis involves innate and acquired immunity. Two major cellular participants in the immune response, macrophages and T lymphocytes, undergo activation in atheroma [59]. The antigenic substances may include oxidized lipoproteins and some stress proteins such as heat shock protein-60. The effector cells of acquired immunity *par excellence*, the CD8-positive T cells, can kill cells by apoptosis via production of perforin, granzyme, and Fas ligand [53]. However, mediators of innate immunity may also contribute to this process. For example, exposure of human SMC to a 'cocktail' of cytokines found in human atheroma, including interleukin-1β (IL-1β), tumor necrosis factor-α (TNF-α), and IFN-γ, can induce apoptosis [7]. In addition, 'priming' of SMC with cytokines implicated in innate immunity can sensitize them to killing by Fas engagement [8]. Thus, the effector limbs of innate and acquired immunity may cooperate in causing the demise of cells within atheroma.

Table 2. Vascular cell apoptosis: Extracellular triggers and inhibitors

Triggers	*References*
OxLDL	41,58,111-113
Oxysterols	47,56,114
Reactive oxygen species	36,44,76
Reactive nitrogen species (NO at high levels)	44
Radiations	38,40,84,115,116
Cytokines	7,8,45,117
Viral and bacterial products	104,105,118
Inhibitors	
Shear stress	31-35
NO at low levels	66,119
PDGF	10,120
VEGF	75,121
bFGF	81,122,123
IGF-I	124
Cowpox virus CrmA	125
Baculovirus protein *p35*	126
The IAP protein family	127,128
Vitamins C and C	52,77,129
Antioxidant enzymes (e.g., SOD and Catalase)	36,43,86,87

The cytokines produced by activated macrophages and T cells can synergistically induce activation of the sphingomyelin-ceramide signaling pathway [60,61] as well as the L-arginine-nitric oxide (NO) pathway, [7,45,62-65] both of which participate in regulation of proliferation as well as apoptosis in vascular SMC. Hence, pro-inflammatory cytokines have overlapping biological effects on vascular cell proliferation and death. When combined, they can exhibit synergy in promoting new gene transcription, e.g., the expression of inducible nitric oxide synthase [63]. This high-capacity isoform of the NO-synthesizing enzyme produces large amounts of NO, a gaseous free radical with multiple biological effects. At high concentrations, NO can attack several important iron-containing enzymes involved in

DNA synthesis and mitochondrial respiration, leading to apoptosis of the target cells. [63, 65] NO can react with superoxide anion (O_2^-) to form the cytotoxic species peroxynitrite ($ONOO^-$), augmenting NO's proapoptotic action [44]. The NO-sensitive iron-containing enzymes in mitochondria include complex I and complex II in the respiratory chain. Since mitochondrial dysfunction critically influences the development of apoptosis (see below), the nitrosylation of iron-enzymes may not only inhibit ATP synthesis but also trigger an apoptotic cascade. The pro-apoptotic effect of NO highly depends upon its concentrations and interactions with other reactive species. Small, physiological amounts of NO show no harm, and under certain circumstances, protective effects against vascular cell apoptosis [32,66,67].

In addition to TNF itself, other members of the TNF superfamily can play important roles in regulation of apoptosis. The fascinating death-signaling protein, Fas/apo-1/CD95, a cell surface-borne protein, belongs to the TNF receptor superfamily. Ligation of Fas by Fas ligand (FasL) or agonistic anti-Fas antibodies can induce apoptosis in activated T lymphocytes. [68] Analysis of markers for apoptosis indicates that many T lymphocytes may undergo apoptosis after they infiltrate atherosclerotic lesions. [69] Several lines of evidence implicate the FasL/Fas-caspase death pathway in induction of apoptosis in atherosclerotic plaques. [8,70,71] The inflammatory cells and vascular cells such as SMC and EC express Fas in atheroma. Although vascular SMC express Fas, the cells do not undergo apoptosis under usual conditions, even in the presence of FasL or agonistic antibodies. [8] However, after pretreatment of SMC with the cytokines TNF-α, IL-1 and IFN-γ, Fas ligation significantly reduces viability and increases internucleosomal DNA fragmentation. Moreover, priming with these cytokines may enhance expression of Fas and provide additional death-promoting signals for initiation or acceleration of the apoptotic cascade in plaque cells. The T lymphocytes in turn (particularly $CD8^+$ cells present in plaques, although less abundant than $CD4^+$ cells) produce effector molecules such as FasL, granzymes and perforin that can kill other plaque cells by apoptosis.

Interestingly, under certain conditions, vascular cells can also express the ligand for Fas, and may thus themselves become triggers for apoptosis. [72] The increased expression of FasL in EC and SMC may trigger apoptosis of 'preemptively' cytotoxic T cells and macrophages and thereby prolong survival of the vascular cells. This mechanism might explain the recent report that overexpression of FasL in the rabbit arteries with hyperlipidemia promotes the development of atherosclerosis, as a result of intimal SMC accumulation [73]. Schaub et al. [74] found that signals initiated by regulated Fas-associated death domain protein overexpression in rat vascular SMC induce expression of monocyte-chemoattractant protein-1 and interleukin-8, and cause massive immigration of macrophages *in vivo*. Chemokines and other pro-inflammatory genes in human vascular SMC elicit expression of a range of Fas-induced apoptosis, in part through a process that requires IL-1 activation. Thus, apoptotic vascular cells may induce proinflammatory responses and contribute to the pathogenesis of vascular disease.

ANTI-APOPTOTIC FACTORS IN ATHEROSCLEROSIS

The regulation of apoptosis involves negative as well as positive signaling. Inhibitors of apoptosis relevant to atherosclerosis include shear stress [33], growth factors [13,75], antioxidant drugs or enzymes (e.g. SOD [76]), and pharmacological doses of antioxidant vitamins, such as vitamin-C and vitamin-E [77] (Table 2). By counteracting the apoptotic effects of cytotoxic factors, these inhibitors may maintain integrity of the endothelium, and increase cellularity of the vessel wall. Mechanical force generated by blood flow can affect endothelial functions and the structure of the vessel wall. Laminar shear stress found in normal arteries can inhibit apoptosis of human EC. [31,66] By contrast, lack of normal shear stress, or in regions of flow disturbances characteristic of sites of predilection to atheroma, may induce apoptosis of EC. [78] The inhibitory effect of shear stress on apoptosis of EC may relate in part to the increased levels of NO produced by the low capacity endothelial isoform of NO synthase, a shear stress-activated gene. In contrast to cytokine-induced NO synthase, constitutive endothelial NOS generates relatively small amounts of NO that may inhibit caspase activities and protect EC from apoptosis. [32,66] Analysis of human atherosclerotic lesions shows more apoptosis in the downstream parts of plaques where disturbed flow occurs. [33] Laminar shear stress can also induce expression of apoptosis-regulating genes in human umbilical vein EC (HUVEC). Bartling et al. [34] applied high levels of laminar shear stress (15 and 30 dyn/cm^2) to human EC. They observed a decreased susceptibility of HUVEC to apoptosis, whereas low shear stress (1 dyn/cm^2) had no effect. These diminished signs of apoptosis occurred in tandem with decreased mRNA expression of apoptosis-inducing Fas. Furthermore, high levels of shear stress induced mRNA and protein expression of anti-apoptotic, soluble Fas isoform FasExo6Del and anti-apoptotic Bcl-x(L). Shear stress also induces Bcl-x(L) and Bak mRNA, counteracted by inhibition of the endothelial NO synthase.

Much of the early work on growth factors such as PDGF and M-CSF focused on their pro-proliferative actions. However, in the context of contemporary apoptosis research, it has become clear that these factors may act as 'survival' factors rather than mediators of mitosis. [79] For example, macrophages deprived of M-CSF will undergo apoptosis induced by denatured, aggregated LDL. [80] Likewise, PDGF protects SMC from apoptosis. [79] Vascular endothelial cell growth factor (VEGF) can inhibit apoptosis of bone marrow cells induced by radiation. [75] Basic fibroblast growth factor (bFGF) can inhibit apoptosis of EC induced by TNF-α. Attenuation of bFGF expression on antisense strategy can trigger apoptosis of vascular SMC. [81] This growth factor also prevents apoptosis induced by serum starvation. [82-84] Protein kinase-C may mediate this protective effect of fibroblast growth factor.

Because oxidative stress can injure vascular cells and promote apoptosis as stated above, antioxidants might mitigate this process. For instance, during 7-ketocholesterol-induced apoptosis of U937 cells, the content of cellular antioxidants falls rapidly [85]. Administration of two potent antioxidants, the aminothiols glutathione (GSH) and N-acetylcysteine (NAC), can protect the monocytic cells from 7-ketocholesterol-induced apoptotic cell death. [85] In addition, some enzymes with the antioxidant properties such as superoxide dismutase (SOD) [86] have been shown to exert protective effects against endothelial apoptosis induced by oxidized lipoproteins. Another antioxidant enzyme catalase was reported to prevent vascular SMC apoptosis triggered by hydrogen peroxide [87]. However, in this report, the authors found that superoxide anion stimulates proliferation rather than induces apoptosis in SMC, which can be blocked by SOD. Thus, different radical species may exert different effects on different cell types.

The interplay of these mitogenic, death-inducing, and survival-promoting factors probably occurs over many years in the history of a given human atherosclerotic lesion. Death of macrophages may lead to accumulation of extracellular lipid and cellular detritus in the 'necrotic core' of the lipid-rich atheroma. Death and disappearance of macrophages and SMC may account for their virtual absence in certain highly fibrotic and calcified late atherosclerotic lesions. The variety of atherosclerotic lesions, even those residing as neighbors within a given human coronary artery, may result from the outcome of this sustained 'tug of war' between cellular death and procreation.

THE CELLULAR METABOLIC PATHWAYS FOR INITIATION AND EXECUTION OF APOPTOSIS

Many surface receptors and intracellular proteins or enzyme systems participate in regulation of apoptosis. Table 3 lists some of these receptors and cellular proteins potentially important for regulation of vascular cell apoptosis during atherogenesis.

Caspases

The cytoplasm contains members of a family of aspartate-specific cysteinyl proteases known as caspases. [88] All members of the caspase family (Table 3), which now number 14, show a similar substrate cleavage at an aspartyl residue and require processing of a zymogen to attain activity. The caspase family participates in downstream events of death signaling by the members of TNF receptor superfamily (e.g., Fas and TNF receptor-1) that share a related intracellular "death domain" of about 70 amino acid residues. The Fas-associated protein with death domain (FADD)/MORT1 and receptor-interacting protein (RIP) and TNFR-1-associated death domain protein (TRADD) serve as downstream messengers in the pathway of apoptosis. Based upon their functions, caspases fall into three groups: (1) those that have a limited role in apoptosis and participate mainly in inflammation (caspases 1, 4, 5, and 11-14); (2) those that serve as initiators of apoptosis (caspases 2 and 8-10); and (3) those that act as effectors of apopotsis (caspases 3, 6, and 7).

Table 3. Cellular functional protein families with the potential of regulating vascular cell apoptosis during atherogenesis

Death receptors	Other names	Ligand
DR3	Apo3, Wsl1, TRAMP, LARD	TWEAK
DR4	Apo2, Trail-R1	Trail
DR5	Trail-R2, TRICK2	Trail
Fas	CD95, Apo1	FasL (CD95L)
TNFR1		TNF
Caspases	**Other names**	**Function**
Caspase-1	ICE	Pro-inflammatory
Caspase-2	ICH-1	Pro-apoptotic
Caspase-3	CPP32, YAMA, Apopain	Pro-apoptotic
Caspase-4	ICErel II, TX, ICH-2	Pro-inflammatory
Caspase-5	ICErel III, TY	Pro-inflammatory
Caspase-6	Mch2	Pro-apoptotic
Caspase-7	Mch3, ICE-LAP3, CMH-1	Pro-apoptotic
Caspase-8	FLICE, MACH, Mch5	Pro-apoptotic
Caspase-9	ICE-Lap6, Mch6, APAF-3	Pro-apoptotic
Caspase-10	Mch4	Pro-apoptotic
Caspase-11		Pro-inflammatory
Caspase-12		Pro-inflammatory
Caspase-13		Pro-inflammatory?
Caspase-14	MICE	Pro-inflammatory/ Pro-apoptotic?

Mitochondrial Bcl2 Family

Pro-apoptotic members

Bad, Bak, Bax, Bcl-Xs, Bid, Bik, Bim, Bod, Bod, Bok, DP5, Hrk, Mtd, Nip3

Anti-apoptotic members

Bcl-2, Bcl-w, Bfl-1, BHRF-1, Boo, Mcl-1

The precise mechanism by which activation of caspases kills cells remains unclear. Available evidence largely from the pro-apoptotic cytokine-receptor death-signaling model and the mitochondrial death model indicates two distinct but related pathways in cell death by apoptosis in atherosclerotic lesions (Figure 1). In pathway one, [68] FasL-Fas ligation or TNF-TNF-R engagement trimerizes the receptor, recruits cofactors such as FADD and RIP, and facilitates activation of pro-caspases 8 and 2 by autoproteolysis and oligomerization. Subsequently, proteolytic activation of the effector caspases 3, 6, and 7 results in cleavage of a variety of substrates within cells. In pathway two, various cytotoxic substances may attack mitochondria [89], translocate pro-apoptotic members of the Bcl-2 family to mitochondria, alter voltage-dependent channels in the mitochondrial membrane, and release cytochrome-c. Bridged by the adaptor molecule Apaf-1, cytochrome-c and caspase-9 form a complex, which in turn activates the effector caspases and triggers the caspase cascade. Interestingly, in some cells, caspase-8 activation can also activate the mitochondrial death pathway by cleavage of Bid, a pro-apoptotic member of the Bcl-2 family. Although the two pathways of apoptosis can operate in the same cells, studies suggest that certain cell types may utilize predominantly one or the other mechanism for apoptosis. In general, pathway one is more active than pathway two in the receptor-mediated cell death. Conversely, pathway two is more prominent in death induced by cytotoxic agents.

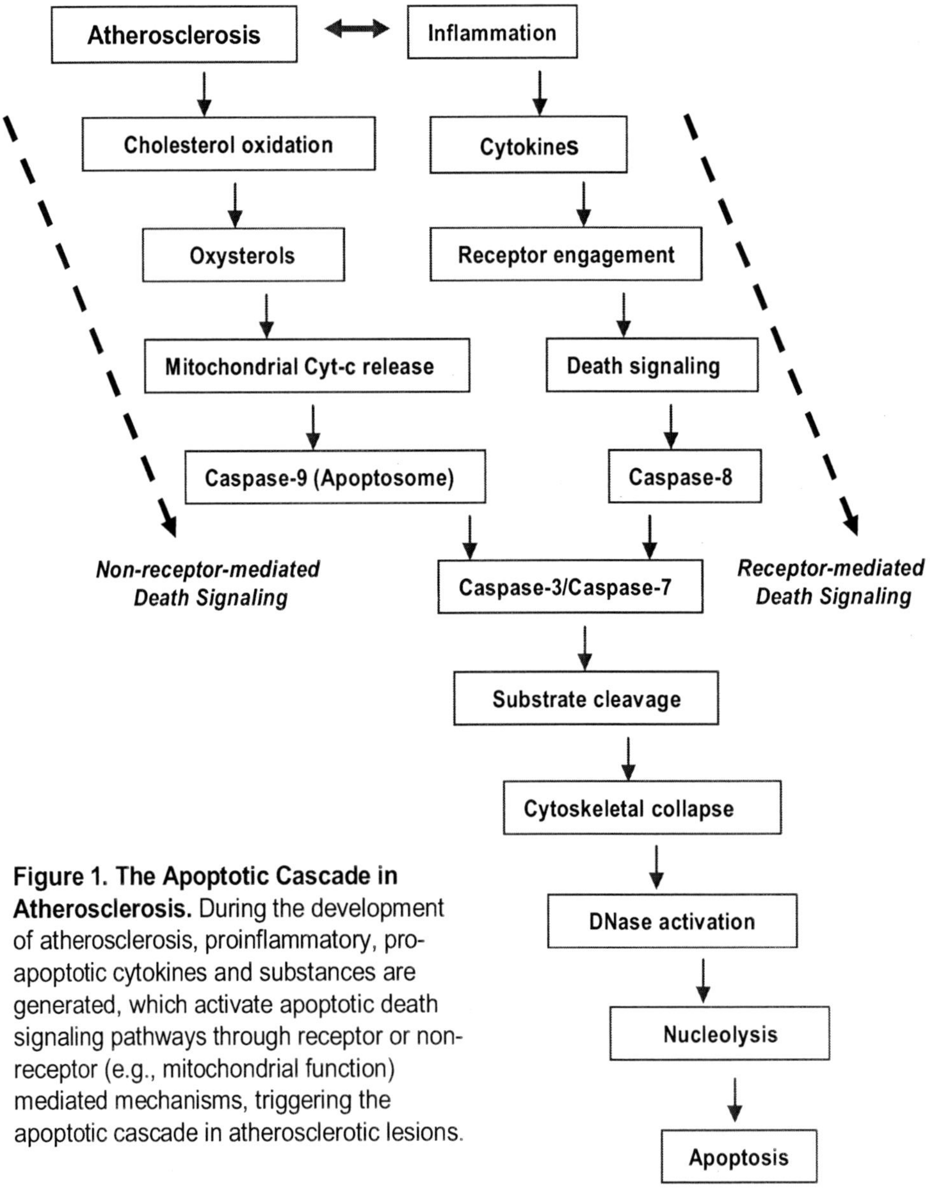

Figure 1. The Apoptotic Cascade in Atherosclerosis. During the development of atherosclerosis, proinflammatory, pro-apoptotic cytokines and substances are generated, which activate apoptotic death signaling pathways through receptor or non-receptor (e.g., mitochondrial function) mediated mechanisms, triggering the apoptotic cascade in atherosclerotic lesions.

Caspases play a critical role in apoptosis of vascular cells in atherosclerotic plaques and in cultured vascular cells [15]. However, the biological functions of caspases in atherosclerotic lesions are largely unknown. Caspases can cleave many intracellular proteins. These substrates include regulators of nuclease activity that play an important role in the final phase of the caspase cascade. Normally, inhibitors of the nucleases protect cells from nucleolysis. Caspase 3 can cleave I^{CAD}/DFF45, an inhibitor of the nuclease responsible for DNA fragmentation, CAD (caspase-activated deoxyribonuclease). [88] In addition, activated caspase 3 also cleaves gelsolin [90,91], an actin-associated protein that may regulate the DNase I activity. In cultured SMC, cytokine-induced activation of caspase 3 triggers an apoptosis cascade in which fragmented gelsolin depolymerizes actin, promotes collapse of cytoskeleton, and induces activation of nucleases that degrade DNA. [91] In human atherosclerosis lesions, increased expression of caspase-3 occurs in both macrophages and smooth muscle cells, and is often associated with apoptotic cells (Figure 2 a and b). In contrast, the arterial media where normal smooth muscle cells reside express little caspase-3 (Figure 2 c). Activated caspase-3 is detectable by immunoblotting with antibodies against the activated form of caspase-3 (Figure 2 d). Caspase-8 or FLICE (Fas-associated death domain-like interleukin 1β-converting enzyme)-inhibitory protein (Flip), a naturally occurring caspase-inhibitory protein that lacks the critical cysteine domain necessary for catalytic activity, negatively regulates Fas-induced apoptosis. [92] During differentiation from monocytes, macrophages can express high levels of FLIP, a potent inhibitor of the caspase 8 activation. [93] During SMC apoptosis, the expression of this protein expression declines.

Bcl-2 and Mitochondria

The Bcl-2 protein family (Table 3) represents another group of cellular proteins that regulate apoptosis in mammalian cells [94]. The mitochondrial membrane contains abundant Bcl-2. [89,94] The Bcl-2 family has more than 15 members. Based upon differences in regulation of apoptosis, members of this family fall into two subgroups. Each of them contains five or more function- and structure-related proteins. The first group includes the anti-apoptotic proteins such as Bcl-2, Bcl-X, Mcl-1, Bcl-w and A1; members of the second group promote apoptosis and include Bax, Bak, Bad, Bik, Hrk, Bid and Bcl-xs. The mechanism by which Bcl-2 inhibits apoptosis remains incompletely clarified. Bcl-2 may exert an antioxidant effect on stressed cells, prevent release of mitochondrial cyto-chrome, and bind to and inactivate pro-apoptotic molecules such as Bax and Bak.

Rapidly accumulating evidence indicates the pivotal role of mitochondria in apoptosis. [89,94] Mitochondria can regulate apoptosis in at least three ways: 1) inhibition of mitochondrial respiration due to production of large amounts of NO in cytokine-stimulated vascular cells [95]; 2) production of cytotoxic reactive oxygen species or change of cellular reduction-oxidation (redox) potential [41,96]; and 3) release of pro-apoptotic molecules including cytochrome-c and apoptosis inducing factor (AIF) [97]. Many Bcl-2 family proteins reside in the mitochondrial outer membrane where they form a pore structure that surprisingly resembles certain bacterial toxins that enhance proton extrusion. The release of cytochrome-c depends on the mitochondrial inner transmembrane potential. When apoptotic stimuli attenuate Bcl-2 function, a rapid drop or collapse of transmembrane potential may occur, causing rapid release of cytochrome-c and other pro-apoptotic proteins. Cytosolic cytochrome-c then forms, together with Apaf-1 and caspase 9, an 'apoptosome' which orchestrates activation of other caspases and distal effectors of apoptosis.

Several groups have recently reported expression of some members of the Bcl-2 protein family in atherosclerosis. [98,99] Although Bcl-2 expression seems controversial, all studies pointed to an imbalance between pro- and anti-apoptotic proteins in the Bcl-2 family. For instance, plaque cells appear to express higher levels of Bax, a pro-apoptotic protein of the Bcl-2 family, than inhibitors such as Bcl-2, indicating an increased activity of pro-apoptotic proteins in the lesions. Regulation of Bcl-2 protein function may be important in vascular cell death. In human endothelial cell apoptosis induced by TNF-α, Bcl-2 specifically undergoes degradation by a process sensitive to proteasome inhibitors. [100] Mutation of the potential ubiquitin-acceptor amino acids of Bcl-2 provides protection against TNF-α and staurosporine-induced Bcl-2 degradation *in vitro* and *in vivo.*

p53 and Oncogenes

Nuclear proteins, particularly those related to oncogenes or anti-oncogenes, [101] such as *p53* and c-*myc*, may also regulate apoptosis of vascular cells during atherogenesis. The tumor suppressor gene *p53* functions as an anti-oncogene capable of promoting apoptosis. Wild-type *p53* arrests cell proliferation and may retain cells with DNA damage in G_1 phase of the cell cycle. During DNA repair, some *p53*-expressing cells oppose the G_1 block and enter the suicide pathway. In atherosclerosis, p53 may mediate apoptosis of vascular cells [102,103]. Mutations in *p53* or its interaction with viral proteins such as simian virus 40 large T antigens or the products of human cytomegalovirus can cause dysfunction of *p53* and, in turn, inhibit apoptosis [104,105]. Cells from normal blood vessels express little *p53*, but vascular cells undergoing apoptosis do contain *p53*. *In vitro* studies furnish further evidence that *p53* regulates apoptosis in cultured SMC. Bennett et al. [106-108] reported that *p53* mediates induction of apoptosis by deprivation of growth factors and transfection with c-*myc* in cultured vascular SMC.

Different oncogenes may interact in the control of apoptosis. Compared with normal cells, SMC from atherosclerotic plaques show a higher ratio of the active (hypophosphorylated) to the inactive (phosphorylated) form of the tumor suppressor gene Rb (retinoblastoma gene product) and a lower level of E2F transcriptional activity. [107] Suppression of RB alone increases rates of cell proliferation and apoptosis and inhibits senescence of normal VSMCs. Suppression of *p53* and RB together exerts similar effects. In contrast, inhibition of RB binding to E2F or ectopic expression of E2F-1 in plaque cells induces massive apoptosis, which requires suppression of *p53* to rescue cells [107]. Suppression of RB and *p53* together increases cell proliferation and delays senescence but fails to immortalize plaque cells. Inhibition of *p53* alone has minimal effect on plaque cells but increases the lifespan of normal SMC.

Arterial injury induces apoptosis as well as proliferation of SMC. Speir et al. [104,105] have presented evidence linking arterial injury, cytomegalovirus, and dysregulated apoptosis.

They reported that some cells in injured arteries could express wild-type *p53*, an inducer of apoptosis. They further observed that human cytomegalovirus binds to and inactivates apoptosis-promoter *p53*, prolonging the life span of SMC. Expression of the human cytomegalovirus protein, IE2-84, but not IE1-72, may protect SMC from *p53*-mediated apoptosis. [105] These observations raise the possibility that attenuation of apoptosis contributes to increased accumulation of cells in the intima and thus to intimal expansion post-arterial injury.

Using compound mutant mice, Guevara, et al. [109] examined the effect of p53 inactivation on atherogenesis in hyperlipidemic apoE-deficient mice. Compared with $p53^{+/+}/apoE^{-/-}$ mice, $p53^{-/-}/apoE^{-/-}$ mice developed accelerated aortic atherosclerosis in place of a similar serum cholesterol levels in response to a high-fat diet. Furthermore, the atherosclerotic lesions in $p53^{-/-}/apoE^{-/-}$ mice had a significant increase in cell proliferation and an insignificant increase in apoptosis compared with those in $p53^{+/+}/apoE^{-/-}$ mice. These observations indicate a role for *p53* in controlling arterial cell replication, suggesting a *p53*-independent mechanism underlying the apoptotic response in this mouse atherosclerosis model.

The proto-oncogene c-*myc* can mediate either cell death or proliferation depending on its level of expression. It functions as a nuclear phosphoprotein with certain properties of a transcription factor. [101] However, in serum-deprived cultures, cells over expressing c-*myc* readily undergo apoptosis. Deregulation of c-*myc* causes apoptosis of the vascular SMC deprived of growth factors or treated with cytokines such as IFN-γ.[110] *p53* may mediate the pro-apoptotic effect of c-*myc* in various cell lines.

Conclusions

Apoptosis probably participates in progression or regression of atherosclerotic lesions, in vascular remodeling, and in complications of advanced atheroma. Many environmental and endogenous factors can influence apoptosis through various signal transduction or enzymatic pathways. The apoptotic mechanisms illustrated above link risk factors (e.g., oxidized lipids) and immune and inflammatory effector mechanisms to disordered cell accumulation, providing a unifying concept situated at the center of current thinking about atherosclerosis. Abnormality of apoptosis may occur in atherosclerosis, favoring accumulation of intimal cells during some phases of atherogenesis. In advanced atheroma, cell death may contribute to aneurysm formation and to weakening of the fibrous cap, enhance thrombogenicity of the lesion's core, and increase the risk of plaque disruption. Future studies will assess whether therapies directed toward apoptosis will modify vascular diseases such as atherosclerosis.

References

[1] Libby P, Clinton SK. Cytokines as mediators of vascular pathology. *Nouv Rev Fr Hematol.* 1992;34:S47-53.

[2] Majno G, Joris I. Apoptosis, oncosis, and necrosis. An overview of cell death. *Am J Pathol.* 1995;146:3-15.

[3] Kockx MM, Muhring J, Bortier H, De MG, Jacob W. Biotin- or digoxigenin-conjugated nucleotides bind to matrix vesicles in atherosclerotic plaques. *Am J Pathol.* 1996;148:1771-7.

[4] Isner JM, Kearney M, Bortman S, Passeri J. Apoptosis in human atherosclerosis and restenosis [see comments]. *Circulation.* 1995;91:2703-11.

[5] Han DK, Haudenschild CC, Hong MK, Tinkle BT, Leon MB, Liau G. Evidence for apoptosis in human atherogenesis and in a rat vascular injury model. *Am J Pathol.* 1995;147:267-77.

[6] Geng YJ, Libby P. Evidence for apoptosis in advanced human atheroma. Colocalization with interleukin-1 beta-converting enzyme. *Am J Pathol.* 1995;147:251-66.

[7] Geng YJ, Wu Q, Muszynski M, Hansson GK, Libby P. Apoptosis of vascular smooth muscle cells induced by in vitro stimulation with interferon-gamma, tumor necrosis factor-alpha, and interleukin-1 beta. *Arterioscler Thromb Vasc Biol.* 1996;16:19-27.

[8] Geng YJ, Henderson LE, Levesque EB, Muszynski M, Libby P. Fas is expressed in human atherosclerotic intima and promotes apoptosis of cytokine-primed human vascular smooth muscle cells. *Arterioscler Thromb Vasc Biol.* 1997;17:2200-8.

[9] Kockx MM, De MG, Muhring J, Bult H, Bultinck J, Herman AG. Distribution of cell replication and apoptosis in atherosclerotic plaques of cholesterol-fed rabbits. *Atherosclerosis.* 1996;120:115-24.

[10] Graf K, Xi XP, Yang D, Fleck E, Hsueh WA, Law RE. Mitogen-activated protein kinase activation is involved in platelet-derived growth factor-directed migration by vascular smooth muscle cells. *Hypertension.* 1997;29:334-9.

[11] Badimon JJ, Fuster V, Chesebro JH, Badimon L. Coronary atherosclerosis. A multifactorial disease. *Circulation.* 1993;87:II3-16.

[12] Fuster V, Badimon JJ, Badimon L. Clinical-pathological correlations of coronary disease progression and regression. *Circulation.* 1992;86:III1-11.

[13] McCaffrey TA, Du B, Fu C, Bray PJ, Sanborn TA, Deutsch E, Tarazona N, Shaknovitch A, Newman G, Patterson C, Bush HL, Jr. The expression of TGF-beta receptors in human atherosclerosis: evidence for acquired resistance to apoptosis due to receptor imbalance. *J Mol Cell Cardiol.* 1999;31:1627-42.

[14] Hansson GK. Immunological control mechanisms in plaque formation. *Basic Res Cardiol.* 1994;89:41-6.

[15] Geng YJ. Biologic effect and molecular regulation of vascular apoptosis in atherosclerosis. *Curr Atheroscler Rep.* 2001;3:234-42.

[16] Liao HS, Kodama T, Geng YJ. Expression of class A scavenger receptor inhibits apoptosis of macrophages triggered by oxidized low density lipoprotein and oxysterol. *Arterioscler Thromb Vasc Biol.* 2000;20:1968-75.

[17] Liao HS, Matsumoto A, Itakura H, Pittman T, Kodama T, Geng YJ. De novo expression of the class-A macrophage scavenger receptor conferring resistance to apoptosis in differentiated human THP-1 monocytic cells. *Cell Death Differ.* 1999;6:245-55.

[18] Kockx MM, De Meyer GR, Muhring J, Jacob W, Bult H, Herman AG. Apoptosis and related proteins in different stages of human atherosclerotic plaques. *Circulation.* 1998;97:2307-15.

[19] Aeschlimann D, Thomazy V. Protein crosslinking in assembly and remodelling of extracellular matrices: the role of transglutaminases. *Connect Tissue Res.* 2000;41:1-27.

[20] Fuster V, Stein B, Ambrose JA, Badimon L, Badimon JJ, Chesebro JH. Atherosclerotic plaque rupture and thrombosis. Evolving concepts. *Circulation.* 1990;82:II47-59.

[21] Libby P, Geng YJ, Sukhova GK, Simon DI, Lee RT. Molecular determinants of atherosclerotic plaque vulnerability. *Ann N Y Acad Sci.* 1997;811:134-42; discussion 142-5.

[22] Libby P, Geng YJ, Aikawa M, Schoenbeck U, Mach F, Clinton SK, Sukhova GK, Lee RT. Macrophages and atherosclerotic plaque stability. *Curr Opin Lipidol.* 1996;7:330-5.

[23] Davies MJ, Woolf N, Rowles P, Richardson PD. Lipid and cellular constituents of unstable human aortic plaques. *Basic Res Cardiol.* 1994;89:33-9.

[24] Golledge J, Greenhalgh RM, Davies AH. The symptomatic carotid plaque. *Stroke.* 2000;31:774-81.

[25] Libby P. Molecular bases of the acute coronary syndromes. *Circulation.* 1995;91:2844-50.

[26] Bombeli T, Karsan A, Tait JF, Harlan JM. Apoptotic vascular endothelial cells become procoagulant. *Blood.* 1997;89:2429-42.

[27] Flynn PD, Byrne CD, Baglin TP, Weissberg PL, Bennett MR. Thrombin generation by apoptotic vascular smooth muscle cells. *Blood.* 1997;89:4378-84.

[28] Greeno EW, Bach RR, Moldow CF. Apoptosis is associated with increased cell surface tissue factor procoagulant activity. *Lab Invest.* 1996;75:281-9.

[29] Holmes DR, Lopez CA, Liao S, Thompson RW. Smooth muscle cell apoptosis and p53 expression in human abdominal aortic aneurysms. *Ann N Y Acad Sci.* 1996;800:286-7.

[30] Henderson EL, Geng Y-J, Sukhova GK, Whittemore AD, Knox J, Libby P. Apoptosis of smooth muscle cells and expression of mediators of cell death by T lymphocytes in human abdominal aortic aneurysms. *Circulation.* 1997;submitted.

[31] Dimmeler S, Haendeler J, Rippmann V, Nehls M, Zeiher AM. Shear stress inhibits apoptosis of human endothelial cells. *Febs Lett.* 1996;399:71-4.

[32] Dimmeler S, Haendeler J, Nehls M, Zeiher AM. Suppression of apoptosis by nitric oxide via inhibition of interleukin-1beta-converting enzyme (ICE)-like and cysteine protease protein (CPP)-32-like proteases. *J Exp Med.* 1997;185:601-7.

[33] Tricot O, Mallat Z, Heymes C, Belmin J, Leseche G, Tedgui A. Relation between endothelial cell apoptosis and blood flow direction in human atherosclerotic plaques. *Circulation.* 2000;101:2450-3.

[34] Bartling B, Tostlebe H, Darmer D, Holtz J, Silber RE, Morawietz H. Shear stress-dependent expression of apoptosis-regulating genes in endothelial cells. *Biochem Biophys Res Commun*. 2000;278:740-6.

[35] Urbich C, Walter DH, Zeiher AM, Dimmeler S. Laminar shear stress upregulates integrin expression: role in endothelial cell adhesion and apoptosis. *Circ Res*. 2000;87:683-9.

[36] Galle J, Heermeier K, Wanner C. Atherogenic lipoproteins, oxidative stress, and cell death. *Kidney Int Suppl*. 1999;71:S62-5.

[37] Gajdusek CM, Tian H, London S, Zhou D, Rasey J, Mayberg MR. Gamma radiation effect on vascular smooth muscle cells in culture. *Int J Radiat Oncol Biol Phys*. 1996;36:821-8.

[38] Langley RE, Bump EA, Quartuccio SG, Medeiros D, Braunhut SJ. Radiation-induced apoptosis in microvascular endothelial cells. *Br J Cancer*. 1997;75:666-72.

[39] Lopez-Candales A, Holmes DR, Scott MJ, Thompson RW, Wickline SA. Effects of ultraviolet light in vascular cells in vitro and in intact atherosclerotic explants: potential role of apoptosis in vascular biology. *Biochem Cell Biol*. 1996;74:333-45.

[40] Verin V, Popowski Y, Bochaton-Piallat ML, Belenger J, Urban P, Neuville P, Redard M, Costa M, Celetta G, Gabbiani G. Intraarterial beta irradiation induces smooth muscle cell apoptosis and reduces medial cellularity in a hypercholesterolemic rabbit restenosis model. *Int J Radiat Oncol Biol Phys*. 2000;46:661-70.

[41] Hsieh C, Yen M, Yen C, Lau Y. Oxidized low density lipoprotein induces apoptosis via generation of reactive oxygen species in vascular smooth muscle cells. *Cardiovasc Res*. 2001;49:135-145.

[42] Johnson TM, Yu ZX, Ferrans VJ, Lowenstein RA, Finkel T. Reactive oxygen species are downstream mediators of p53- dependent apoptosis. *Proc Natl Acad Sci U S A*. 1996;93:11848-52.

[43] Li PF, Dietz R, von HR. Reactive oxygen species induce apoptosis of vascular smooth muscle cell. *Febs Lett*. 1997;404:249-52.

[44] Patel RP, Moellering D, Murphy-Ullrich J, Jo H, Beckman JS, Darley-Usmar VM. Cell signaling by reactive nitrogen and oxygen species in atherosclerosis. *Free Radic Biol Med*. 2000;28:1780-94.

[45] Geng YJ, Hellstrand K, Wennmalm A, Hansson GK. Apoptotic death of human leukemic cells induced by vascular cells expressing nitric oxide synthase in response to gamma- interferon and tumor necrosis factor-alpha. *Cancer Res*. 1996;56:866-74.

[46] Nishio E, Watanabe Y. Oxysterols induced apoptosis in cultured smooth muscle cells through CPP32 protease activation and bcl-2 protein downregulation. *Biochem Biophys Res Commun*. 1996;226:928-34.

[47] Thompson EB, Ayala-Torres S. Oxysterols and apoptosis: evidence for gene regulation outside the cholesterol pathway. *Crit Rev Biochem Mol Biol*. 1999;34:25-32.

[48] Harada-Shiba M, Kinoshita M, Kamido H, Shimokado K. Oxidized low density lipoprotein induces apoptosis in cultured human umbilical vein endothelial cells by common and unique mechanisms. *J Biol Chem*. 1998;273:9681-7.

[49] Kovacs A, Weber ML, Burns LJ, Jacob HS, Vercellotti GM. Cytoplasmic sequestration of p53 in cytomegalovirus-infected human endothelial cells. *Am J Pathol.* 1996;149:1531-9.

[50] Eldor A, Sela DD, Korner M, Pick M, Resnick RN, Panet A. Injury models of the vascular endothelium: apoptosis and loss of thromboresistance induced by a viral protein. *Haemostasis*. 1996:37-45.

[51] Sela DD, Korner M, Pick M, Eldor A, Panet A. Programmed endothelial cell death induced by an avian hemangioma retrovirus is density dependent. *Virology.* 1996;223:233-7.

[52] Haendeler J, Zeiher AM, Dimmeler S. Vitamin C and E prevent lipopolysaccharide-induced apoptosis in human endothelial cells by modulation of Bcl-2 and Bax. *Eur J Pharmacol.* 1996;317:407-11.

[53] Henderson EL, Geng YJ, Sukhova GK, Whittemore AD, Knox J, Libby P. Death of smooth muscle cells and expression of mediators of apoptosis by T lymphocytes in human abdominal aortic aneurysms. *Circulation.* 1999;99:96-104.

[54] Obara H, Takayanagi A, Hirahashi J, Tanaka K, Wakabayashi G, Matsumoto K, Shimazu M, Shimizu N, Kitajima M. Overexpression of truncated IkappaBalpha induces TNF-alpha-dependent apoptosis in human vascular smooth muscle cells. *Arterioscler Thromb Vasc Biol.* 2000;20:2198-204.

[55] Kellner-Weibel G, Geng YJ, Rothblat GH. Cytotoxic cholesterol is generated by the hydrolysis of cytoplasmic cholesteryl ester and transported to the plasma membrane. *Atherosclerosis*. 1999;146:309-19.

[56] Brown AJ, Jessup W. Oxysterols and atherosclerosis. *Atherosclerosis*. 1999;142:1-28.

[57] Escargueil-Blanc I, Andrieu-Abadie N, Caspar-Bauguil S, Brossmer R, Levade T, Negre-Salvayre A, Salvayre R. Apoptosis and activation of the sphingomyelin-ceramide pathway induced by oxidized low density lipoproteins are not causally related in ECV-304 endothelial cells. *J Biol Chem*. 1998;273:27389-95.

[58] Heermeier K, Leicht W, Palmetshofer A, Ullrich M, Wanner C, Galle J. Oxidized LDL Suppresses NF-kappaB and Overcomes Protection from Apoptosis in Activated Endothelial Cells. *J Am Soc Nephrol*. 2001;12:456-463.

[59] Libby P, Hansson GK. Involvement of the immune system in human atherogenesis: current knowledge and unanswered questions. *Lab Invest*. 1991;64:5-15.

[60] Auge N, Negre-Salvayre A, Salvayre R, Levade T. Sphingomyelin metabolites in vascular cell signaling and atherogenesis. *Prog Lipid Res*. 2000;39:207-29.

[61] Chatterjee S. Sphingolipids in atherosclerosis and vascular biology. *Arterioscler Thromb Vasc Biol*. 1998;18:1523-33.

[62] Hansson GK, Geng YJ, Holm J, Hardhammar P, Wennmalm A, Jennische E. Arterial smooth muscle cells express nitric oxide synthase in response to endothelial injury. *J Exp Med*. 1994;180:733-8.

[63] Geng Y, Hansson GK, Holme E. Interferon-gamma and tumor necrosis factor synergize to induce nitric oxide production and inhibit mitochondrial respiration in vascular smooth muscle cells. *Circ Res*. 1992;71:1268-76.

[64] Geng YJ, Almqvist M, Hansson GK. cDNA cloning and expression of inducible nitric oxide synthase from rat vascular smooth muscle cells. *Biochim Biophys Acta.* 1994;1218:421-4.

[65] Geng YJ, Petersson AS, Wennmalm A, Hansson GK. Cytokine-induced expression of nitric oxide synthase results in nitrosylation of heme and nonheme iron proteins in vascular smooth muscle cells. *Exp Cell Res*. 1994;214:418-28.

[66] Dimmeler S, Zeiher AM. Nitric oxide-an endothelial cell survival factor. *Cell Death Differ*. 1999;6:964-8.

[67] Dimmeler S, Rippmann V, Weiland U, Haendeler J, Zeiher AM. Angiotensin II induces apoptosis of human endothelial cells. Protective effect of nitric oxide. *Circ Res*. 1997;81:970-6.

[68] Ashkenazi A, Dixit VM. Death receptors: signaling and modulation. *Science.* 1998;281:1305-8.

[69] Bjorkerud S, Bjorkerud B. Apoptosis is abundant in human atherosclerotic lesions, especially in inflammatory cells (macrophages and T cells), and may contribute to the accumulation of gruel and plaque instability. *Am J Pathol*. 1996;149:367-80.

[70] Cai W, Devaux B, Schaper W, Schaper J. The role of Fas/APO 1 and apoptosis in the development of human atherosclerotic lesions [In Process Citation]. *Atherosclerosis*. 1997;131:177-86.

[71] Fukuo K, Nakahashi T, Nomura S, Hata S, Suhara T, Shimizu M, Tamatani M, Morimoto S, Kitamura Y, Ogihara T. Possible participation of Fas-mediated apoptosis in the mechanism of atherosclerosis. *Gerontology*. 1997;1:35-42.

[72] Walsh K, Sata M. Is extravasation a Fas-regulated process? *Mol Med Today*. 1999;5:61-7.

[73] Schneider DB, Vassalli G, Wen S, Driscoll RM, Sassani AB, DeYoung MB, Linnemann R, Virmani R, Dichek DA. Expression of Fas ligand in arteries of hypercholesterolemic rabbits accelerates atherosclerotic lesion formation. *Arterioscler Thromb Vasc Biol*. 2000;20:298-308.

[74] Schaub FJ, Han DK, Liles WC, Adams LD, Coats SA, Ramachandran RK, Seifert RA, Schwartz SM, Bowen-Pope DF. Fas/FADD-mediated activation of a specific program of inflammatory gene expression in vascular smooth muscle cells. *Nat Med*. 2000;6:790-6.

[75] Katoh O, Tauchi H, Kawaishi K, Kimura A, Satow Y. Expression of the vascular endothelial growth factor (VEGF) effect of VEGF on apoptotic cell death caused by ionizing radiation. *Cancer Res*. 1995;55:5687-92.

[76] Heermeier K, Schneider R, Heinloth A, Wanner C, Dimmeler S, Galle J. Oxidative stress mediates apoptosis induced by oxidized low-density lipoprotein and oxidized lipoprotein(a). *Kidney Int*. 1999;56:1310-2.

[77] Siow RC, Sato H, Leake DS, Ishii T, Bannai S, Mann GE. Induction of antioxidant stress proteins in vascular endothelial and smooth muscle cells: protective action of vitamin C against atherogenic lipoproteins. *Free Radic Res*. 1999;31:309-18.

[78] Kaiser D, Freyberg MA, Friedl P. Lack of hemodynamic forces triggers apoptosis in vascular endothelial cells. *Biochem Biophys Res Commun*. 1997;231:586-90.

[79] Bennett MR, Evan GI, Schwartz SM. Apoptosis of human vascular smooth muscle cells derived from normal vessels and coronary atherosclerotic plaques. *J Clin Invest.* 1995;95:2266-74.

[80] Kubo N, Kikuchi J, Furukawa Y, Sakai T, Ohta H, Iwase S, Yamada H, Sakurabayashi I. Regulatory effects of aggregated LDL on apoptosis during foam cell formation of human peripheral blood monocytes. *Febs Lett.* 1997;409:177-82.

[81] Fox JC, Shanley JR. Antisense inhibition of basic fibroblast growth factor induces apoptosis in vascular smooth muscle cells. *J Biol Chem.* 1996;271:12578-84.

[82] Araki S, Simada Y, Kaji K, Hayashi H. Role of protein kinase C in the inhibition by fibroblast growth factor of apoptosis in serum-depleted endothelial cells. *Biochem Biophys Res Commun.* 1990;172:1081-5.

[83] Kondo S, Yin D, Aoki T, Takahashi JA, Morimura T, Takeuchi J. bcl-2 gene prevents apoptosis of basic fibroblast growth factor- deprived murine aortic endothelial cells. *Exp Cell Res.* 1994;213:428-32.

[84] Haimovitz FA, Balaban N, McLoughlin M, Ehleiter D, Michaeli J, Vlodavsky I, Fuks Z. Protein kinase C mediates basic fibroblast growth factor protection of endothelial cells against radiation-induced apoptosis. *Cancer Res.* 1994;54:2591-7.

[85] Lizard G, Gueldry S, Sordet O, Monier S, Athias A, Miguet C, Bessede G, Lemaire S, Solary E, Gambert P. Glutathione is implied in the control of 7-ketocholesterol-induced apoptosis, which is associated with radical oxygen species production. *Faseb J.* 1998;12:1651-63.

[86] Yokoyama I, Negita M, Hayakawa A, Takebe A, Hayashi S, Kobayashi T, Katayama A, Namii Y, Nagasaka T, Koike C, Kojima T, Takagi, H. Apoptosis in pig endothelial cells after reperfusion and its prevention by genetic induction of human Cu, Zn-SOD cDNA. *Transplant Proc.* 1997;2:1364.

[87] Li PF, Dietz R, von Harsdorf R. Differential effect of hydrogen peroxide and superoxide anion on apoptosis and proliferation of vascular smooth muscle cells. *Circulation.* 1997;96:3602-9.

[88] Thornberry NA, Lazebnik Y. Caspases: enemies within. *Science.* 1998;281:1312-6.

[89] Green DR, Reed JC. Mitochondria and apoptosis. *Science.* 1998;281:1309-12.

[90] Kothakota S, Azuma T, Reinhard C, Klippel A, Tang J, Chu K, McGarry TJ, Kirschner MW, Koths K, Kwiatkowski DJ, Williams LT. Caspase-3-generated fragment of gelsolin: effector of morphological change in apoptosis. *Science.* 1997;278:294-8.

[91] Geng YJ, Azuma T, Tang JX, Hartwig JH, Muszynski M, Wu Q, Libby P, Kwiatkowski DJ. Caspase-3-induced gelsolin fragmentation contributes to actin cytoskeletal collapse, nucleolysis, and apoptosis of vascular smooth muscle cells exposed to proinflammatory cytokines. *Eur J Cell Biol.* 1998;77:294-302.

[92] Irmler M, Thome M, Hahne M, Schneider P, Hofmann K, Steiner V, Bodmer JL, Schroter M, Burns K, Mattmann C, Rimoldi D, French LE, Tschopp J. Inhibition of death receptor signals by cellular FLIP [see comments]. *Nature.* 1997;388:190-5.

[93] Perlman H, Pagliari LJ, Georganas C, Mano T, Walsh K, Pope RM. FLICE-inhibitory protein expression during macrophage differentiation confers resistance to fas-mediated apoptosis. *J Exp Med.* 1999;190:1679-88.

[94] Adams JM, Cory S. The Bcl-2 protein family: arbiters of cell survival. *Science.* 1998;281:1322-6.

[95] Geng YJ. Molecular signal transduction in vascular cell apoptosis. *Cell Res.* 2001;11:253-64.

[96] Dimmeler S, Zeiher AM. Reactive oxygen species and vascular cell apoptosis in response to angiotensin II and pro-atherosclerotic factors. *Regul Pept.* 2000;90:19-25.

[97] Susin SA, Lorenzo HK, Zamzami N, Marzo I, Snow BE, Brothers GM, Mangion J, Jacotot E, Costantini P, Loeffler M, Larochette N, Goodlett DR, Aebersold R, Siderovski DP, Penninger JM, Kroemer G. Molecular characterization of mitochondrial apoptosis-inducing factor [see comments]. *Nature.* 1999;397:441-6.

[98] Hayakawa Y, Takemura G, Misao J, Kanoh M, Ohno M, Ohashi H, Takatsu H, Ito H, Fukuda K, Fujiwara T, Minatoguchi S, Fujiwara H. Apoptosis and overexpression of bax protein and bax mRNA in smooth muscle cells within intimal hyperplasia of human radial arteries : analysis with arteriovenous fistulas used for hemodialysis. *Arterioscler Thromb Vasc Biol.* 1999;19:2066-77.

[99] Saxena A, McMeekin JD, Thomson DJ. Expression of Bcl-x, Bcl-2, Bax, and Bak in endarterectomy and atherectomy specimens. *J Pathol.* 2002;196:335-42.

[100] Dimmeler S, Breitschopf K, Haendeler J, Zeiher AM. Dephosphorylation targets Bcl-2 for ubiquitin-dependent degradation: a link between the apoptosome and the proteasome pathway. *J Exp Med.* 1999;189:1815-22.

[101] Evan G, Littlewood T. A matter of life and cell death. *Science.* 1998;281:1317-22.

[102] Ihling C, Haendeler J, Menzel G, Hess RD, Fraedrich G, Schaefer HE, Zeiher AM. Co-expression of p53 and MDM2 in human atherosclerosis: implications for the regulation of cellularity of atherosclerotic lesions. *J Pathol.* 1998;185:303-12.

[103] Aoki M, Morishita R, Matsushita H, Nakano N, Hayashi S, Tomita N, Yamamoto K, Moriguchi A, Higaki J, Ogihara T. Serum deprivation-induced apoptosis accompanied by up-regulation of p53 and bax in human aortic vascular smooth muscle cells. *Heart Vessels.* 1997;Suppl:71-5.

[104] Speir E, Huang ES, Modali R, Leon MB, Shawl F, Finkel T, Epstein SE. Interaction of human cytomegalovirus with p53: possible role in coronary restenosis. *Scand J Infect Dis Suppl.* 1995;99:78-81.

[105] Tanaka K, Zou JP, Takeda K, Ferrans VJ, Sandford GR, Johnson TM, Finkel T, Epstein SE. Effects of human cytomegalovirus immediate-early proteins on p53-mediated apoptosis in coronary artery smooth muscle cells. *Circulation.* 1999;99:1656-9.

[106] Bennett MR, Evan GI, Schwartz SM. Apoptosis of rat vascular smooth muscle cells is regulated by p53- dependent and -independent pathways. *Circ Res.* 1995;77:266-73.

[107] Bennett MR, Macdonald K, Chan SW, Boyle JJ, Weissberg PL. Cooperative interactions between RB and p53 regulate cell proliferation, cell senescence, and apoptosis in human vascular smooth muscle cells from atherosclerotic plaques. *Circ Res.* 1998;82:704-12.

[108] Bennett MR, Littlewood TD, Schwartz SM, Weissberg PL. Increased sensitivity of human vascular smooth muscle cells from atherosclerotic plaques to p53-mediated apoptosis. *Circ Res.* 1997;81:591-9.

[109] Guevara NV, Kim HS, Antonova EI, Chan L. The absence of p53 accelerates atherosclerosis by increasing cell proliferation in vivo. *Nat Med.* 1999;5:335-9.

[110] Bennett MR, Evan GI, Newby AC. Deregulated expression of the c-myc oncogene abolishes inhibition of proliferation of rat vascular smooth muscle cells by serum reduction, interferon-gamma, heparin, and cyclic nucleotide analogues and induces apoptosis. *Circ Res.* 1994;74:525-36.

[111] Nishio E, Arimura S, Watanabe Y. Oxidized LDL induces apoptosis in cultured smooth muscle cells: a possible role for 7-ketocholesterol. *Biochem Biophys Res Commun.* 1996;223:413-8.

[112] Vieira O, Escargueil-Blanc I, Jurgens G, Borner C, Almeida L, Salvayre R, Negre-Salvayre A. Oxidized LDLs alter the activity of the ubiquitin-proteasome pathway: potential role in oxidized LDL-induced apoptosis. *Faseb J.* 2000;14:532-42.

[113] Okura Y, Brink M, Itabe H, Scheidegger KJ, Kalangos A, Delafontaine P. Oxidized Low-Density Lipoprotein Is Associated With Apoptosis of Vascular Smooth Muscle Cells in Human Atherosclerotic Plaques. *Circulation.* 2000;102:2680-2686.

[114] Schroepfer GJ, Jr. Oxysterols: modulators of cholesterol metabolism and other processes. *Physiol Rev.* 2000;80:361-554.

[115] Wilcox JN, Waksman R, King SB, Scott NA. The role of the adventitia in the arterial response to angioplasty: the effect of intravascular radiation. *Int J Radiat Oncol Biol Phys.* 1996;36:789-96.

[116] Kitada S, Krajewski S, Miyashita T, Krajewska M, Reed JC. Gamma-radiation induces upregulation of Bax protein and apoptosis in radiosensitive cells in vivo. *Oncogene.* 1996;12:187-92.

[117] Sato I, Kaji K, Murota S. Age related decline in cytokine induced nitric oxide synthase activation and apoptosis in cultured endothelial cells:. *Mech Ageing Dev.* 1995;81:27-36.

[118] Matturri L, Cazzullo A, Turconi P, Roncoroni L, Grana D, Milei J. Inflammatory cells, apoptosis and chlamydia pneumoniae infection in atherosclerosis. *Int J Cardiol.* 2000;75:23-33.

[119] Jeremy JY, Rowe D, Emsley AM, Newby AC. Nitric oxide and the proliferation of vascular smooth muscle cells. *Cardiovasc Res.* 1999;43:580-94.

[120] Newby AC, George SJ. Proliferation, migration, matrix turnover, and death of smooth muscle cells in native coronary and vein graft atherosclerosis. *Curr Opin Cardiol.* 1996;11:574-82.

[121] Reinmuth N, Liu W, Jung YD, Ahmad SA, Shaheen RM, Fan F, Bucana CD, McMahon G, Gallick GE, Ellis LM. Induction of VEGF in perivascular cells defines a potential paracrine mechanism for endothelial cell survival. *Faseb J.* 2001;15:1239-41.

[122] Miyamoto T, Leconte I, Swain JL, Fox JC. Autocrine FGF signaling is required for vascular smooth muscle cell survival in vitro. *J Cell Physiol.* 1998;177:58-67.

[123] Kondo S, Kondo Y, Yin D, Barnett GH, Kaakaji R, Peterson JW, Morimura T, Kubo H, Takeuchi J, Barna BP. Involvement of interleukin-1 beta-converting enzyme in apoptosis of bFGF-deprived murine aortic endothelial cells. *Faseb J.* 1996;10:1192-7.

[124] Buerke M, Murohara T, Skurk C, Nuss C, Tomaselli K, Lefer AM. Cardioprotective effect of insulin-like growth factor I in myocardial ischemia followed by reperfusion. *Proc Natl Acad Sci U S A*. 1995;92:8031-5.

[125] Tewari M, Quan LT, O'Rourke K, Desnoyers S, Zeng Z, Beidler DR, Poirier GG, Salvesen GS, Dixit VM. Yama/CPP32 beta, a mammalian homolog of CED-3, is a CrmA-inhibitable protease that cleaves the death substrate poly(ADP-ribose) polymerase. *Cell*. 1995;81:801-9.

[126] Datta R, Banach D, Kojima H, Talanian RV, Alnemri ES, Wong WW, Kufe DW. Activation of the CPP32 protease in apoptosis induced by 1-beta-D-arabinofuranosylcytosine and other DNA-damaging agents. *Blood*. 1996;88:1936-43.

[127] Cai W, Devaux B, Schaper W, Schaper J. The role of Fas/APO 1 and apoptosis in the development of human atherosclerotic lesions. *Atherosclerosis*. 1997;131:177-86.

[128] Wang CY, Mayo MW, Korneluk RG, Goeddel DV, Baldwin AS. NF-kappaB antiapoptosis: induction of TRAF1 and TRAF2 and c-IAP1 and c-IAP2 to suppress caspase-8 activation. *Science*. 1998;281:1680-3.

[129] Siow RC, Richards JP, Pedley KC, Leake DS, Mann GE. Vitamin C protects human vascular smooth muscle cells against apoptosis induced by moderately oxidized LDL containing high levels of lipid hydroperoxides. *Arterioscler Thromb Vasc Biol*. 1999;19:2387-94.

ACKNOWLEDGMENTS

This work is supported by grants to Dr. Yong-Jian Geng from NIH (HL59249), Pfizer/Parke-Davis ARA Award, the Fourjay Foundation, and the DREMS program of the Department of Defense.

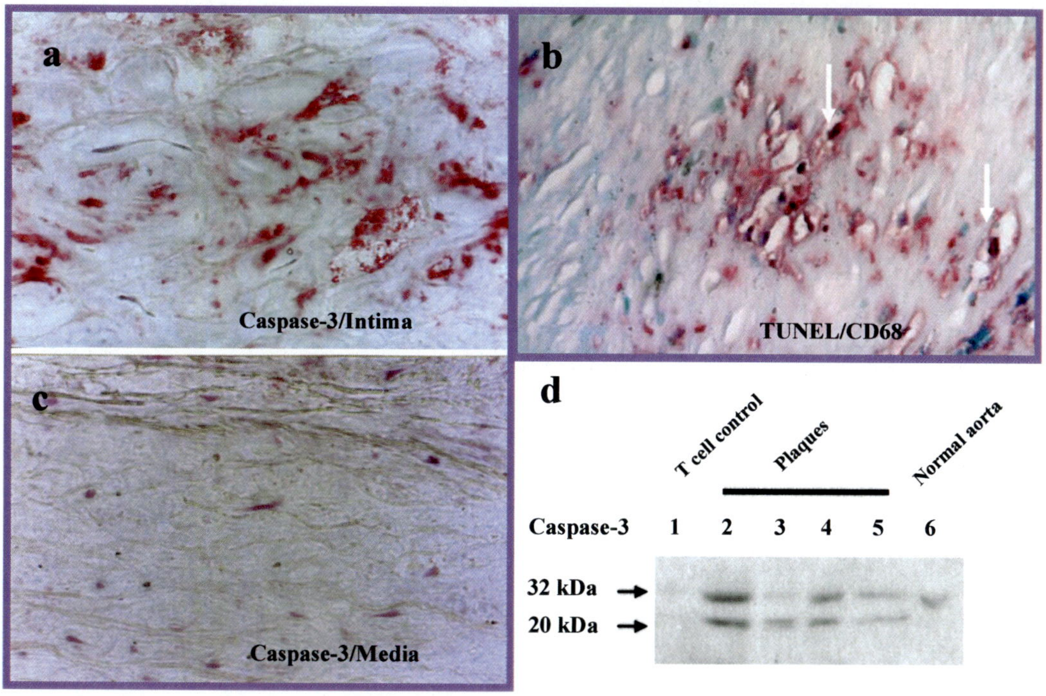

Figure 2. Caspase-3 expression in advanced atherosclerotic lesions or atheroma of human coronary arteries. a, immunostaining for caspase-3 in the intima lesion; b, TUNEL and anti-CD68 staining in a parallel section; c, negative staining for caspase-3 in the media; and d, Western blot analysis showing about 20 kDa activated caspase-3 vs. its pre-enzyme at 32 kDa in the plaque tissue as well as normal aorta and T cells. Images were taken using a 40x objective.

In: Current Topics in Atherosclerosis Research
Editor: Yong J. Geng, pp. 49-65

ISBN 1-59454-428-X

Chapter III

INFLAMMATORY VASCULAR MARKERS IN ATHEROSCLEROSIS

Paolo Calabrò[1] and Edward T.H.Yeh[2,*]

[1]Brown Foundation Institute of Molecular Medicine for the Prevention of Human Diseases, The University of Texas-Houston Health Science Center,
[2]Department of Cardiology, The University of Texas-MD Anderson Cancer Center, Houston, Texas

ABSTRACT

Inflammatory processes of the vascular wall are now recognized to play a central role in the pathogenesis of atherosclerosis. Early atherosclerotic lesion development involves tethering and adherence of monocytes to, and subsequent transmigration through, the vascular endothelium. Differentiation of monocytes to macrophages and subsequent accumulation of lipid results in foam cell generation and fatty streak formation. Further recruitment of inflammatory cells and proliferation of smooth muscle cells lead to the development of a mature atherosclerotic plaque, with a fibrous cap separating the prothrombotic lipid pool from luminal blood flow. Fibrous cap thinning may lead to plaque rupture and precipitate the onset of an acute ischemic event. Accumulating evidence suggests that inflammatory processes are intimately involved in each of these stages in atherogenesis. Plasma levels of several markers of inflammation have been found to be associated with future cardiovascular risk in a variety of clinical settings. These markers include cell adhesion molecules, pro-atherogenic enzymes, cytokines, and C-reactive protein (CRP). The adherence and subsequent transmigration of leukocytes across the vascular endothelium are mediated by cellular adhesion molecules (CAMs). The selectins are adhesion molecules that mediate the initial rolling of inflammatory cells along endothelial cells and platelets. TNF-α is a pleiotropic

* Correspondence concerning this article should be addressed to Professor Edward T.H. Yeh, MD; Department of Cardiology, Unit 449, The University of Texas M. D. Anderson Cancer Center, 1515 Holcombe Blvd., Houston, TX 77030. Telephone: (713) 792-6242. Fax: (713) 745-1942. E-mail: etyeh@mdanderson.org

cytokine produced by a variety of cells including macrophages, endothelial cells, and smooth muscle cells. TNF-α, along with interferon-γ and IL-1, stimulates IL-6 production by smooth muscle cells. IL-6 gene transcripts are expressed in human atheromatous lesions, and this cytokine is the main stimulus for C-reactive protein (CRP) production. Initially thought of as an inactive downstream marker of the inflammatory cascade, emerging evidence suggests that CRP may be directly involved in atherogenesis, and that arterial plaque can produce CRP, independent of traditional hepatic pathways. Finally, other inflammatory markers currently under investigation include some pro-atherogenic enzymes like myeloperoxidase, pregnancy-associated plasma protein A, and lipoprotein-associated phospholipase A_2. The addition of the screening for these new markers of inflammation to traditional lipid testing has the potential to identify individuals at high risk for future cardiovascular events who may benefit from targeted preventive interventions.

Keywords: Inflammation, Atherosclerosis, Cytokines, Adhesion Proteins, C-Reactive Protein

INTRODUCTION

Over the last ten years, our understanding of the role of inflammation in atherosclerosis has flourished. Although it was formerly considered a bland lipid storage disease, substantial advances in basic and experimental science have illuminated the role of inflammation and the underlying cellular and molecular mechanisms that contribute to atherogenesis, leading to current views regard atherosclerosis as a dynamic and progressive disease arising from the combination of endothelial dysfunction and inflammation [1-3].

Inflammatory mechanisms play a central role in mediating all phases of atherosclerosis, from initial recruitment of circulating leukocytes to the arterial wall to the plaque progression, to the eventual rupture of the unstable atherosclerotic plaque [4].

In a variety of animal models of atherosclerosis, signs of inflammation accompany the earliest accumulation of lipid within the artery wall. It is the vascular endothelium, located at the interface of blood and tissue that is able to sense changes in hemodynamic forces and blood borne signals and react by synthesizing and releasing vasoactive substances, maintaining vascular homeostasis. With disruption of this balance, mediated by inflammatory and traditional cardiovascular risk factors, the vasculature becomes susceptible to atheroma formation. Inflammatory mediators appear to play a fundamental role in the initiation, progression, and eventual rupture of atherosclerotic plaques.

As evidence accumulates linking inflammatory processes to atherogenesis, markers of inflammation and endothelial activation may become useful by providing additional information about a patient's risk of developing cardiovascular disease, as well as providing new targets for treatment [5,6].

The Role of the Inflammation in the Atherogenesis

Important works in the 1990s demonstrated that the majority of myocardial infarctions were caused by atherosclerotic coronary lesions resulting in less than 50% luminal obstruction [7,8]. This led to a new evaluation of the type of atheromatous plaque that is prone to precipitate acute ischemic complications: it was now clear that atherosclerotic lesion biology, rather than hydraulics, is the most important determinant of the plaque future [9].

Over the past decade, several experimental evidences have suggested that inflammatory process mediate the initiation and evolution of the atherosclerotic lesion, as well as contributing to the ultimate development of acute coronary syndromes [1]. Circulating leukocytes do not adhere to the normal endothelium. However, when endothelial cells exposed to inflammatory and traditional cardiovascular risk factors undergo inflammatory activation, they begin to express adhesion molecules that selectively bind to circulating leukocytes. These cell adhesion molecules (CAMs) include the selectins [10], P- and E-selectin, and members of the immunoglobulin super family, intercellular adhesion molecule-1 (ICAM-1) and vascular adhesion molecule-1 (VCAM-1) [11]. Adhesion molecule expression is induced by several proinflammatory cytokines such as interleukin-1β (IL-1β) [12], tumor necrosis factor-α (TNF-α) [13], interferon-γ (IFN-γ) [14], by the acute-phase protein C-reactive protein (CRP) [15], by CD40/CD40 ligand interactions [16] and by oxidized low-density lipoprotein (oxLDL) uptake via oxLDL receptor-1 (LOX-1) [17]. The selectins mediate transient rolling of the leukocytes along the endothelium, while stronger attachment is mediated by ICAM-1 and VCAM-1 [18]. Interestingly, knockout mice deficient in E-selectin, P-selectin or ICAM-1 develop less atherosclerosis than normal mice [19,20].

Once adherent to the endothelium, inflammatory cells migrate into the sub-endothelial space, attracted by monocyte chemoattractant protein-1 (MCP-1) [21]. Here, the leucocytes contribute to the local inflammatory response with macrophages expressing receptors like SR-A, CD36, and LOX-1 that internalize modified lipoproteins and macrophage colony stimulating factor combining with MCP-1 to augment the differentiation of blood-derived monocytes into macrophage foam cells [22]. Within the developing atheroma, macrophages, endothelial cells and smooth muscle cells produce the pleiotropic cytokine TNF-α [23], which, together with IFN-γ and IL-1, stimulates smooth muscle cell production of IL-6 [24]; interestingly, IL-6 protein and mRNA has been found in human atheroma [25] and IL-6 is one of the main stimulus for the hepatic and extra-hepatic synthesis of the CRP [26,27]. In particular, we have recently published a direct demonstration that cells present in the arterial wall, like the smooth muscle cells (SMCs), are a source of locally produced CRP [27]. Maximal CRP production, evaluated by a specific ELISA, was observed in SMCs after 48 hours of incubation with the combination of IL-1ß and IL-6, whereas incubation with IL-1ß or IL-6 alone only modestly induced CRP. Incubation with TNF-α or LPS resulted in an increase in CRP production comparable to the IL-1ß and IL-6 combination. Moreover, the induction of CRP in SMCs was independently confirmed by RT-PCR comparing the relative CRP mRNA levels. This locally produced CRP can directly participate in atherogenesis and the development of cardiovascular complications [28]. This acute phase protein indeed has been shown by our group and others to have a direct effect to promote atherosclerotic process and endothelial cell and smooth muscle cell activation [15,29-34]. This local proinflammatory status maintains a chemotactic stimulus for adherent leukocytes, augment the expression of scavenger receptors, and promote further macrophage replication. Another important complex, which plays a critical role in this phase of the inflammation/atherosclerosis process is the CD40 ligand and its receptor CD40 that are expressed by a wide variety of inflammatory cells: ligation of CD40 triggers the expression of a host of proinflammatory mediators such as cytokines, chemokines, ICAM-1 and VCAM-1 [16]. In addition CD40 ligation mediates the expression of matrix metalloproteinases [35], which can breakdown the collagen, as well as tissue factor, an important mediator of thrombosis [36]. In addition to the 39-kDa, cell-associated form, CD40L also occurs in a soluble, biologically fully active form (sCD40L) [37].

If the inflammatory risk factors remain the newly formed atheroma will progress to form a more complex lesion. This process is characterized by the formation of a lipid pool, rich in prothrombotic tissue factor and by the proliferation of smooth muscle cells, their migration toward the intima, and their synthesis of collagen which contributes to the strength of the fibrous cap. The expansion of this lesion within the coronary arteries can result in reduction of the blood flow due to lumen obstruction, clinically represented by the angina. The dynamic balance between the synthesis and the breakdown of collagen in the fibrous cap is regulated by cytokines [9]: indeed, platelet-derived growth factor (PDGF) and transforming growth factor-β (TGF-β) increase the rate of collagen production; conversely, IFN-γ can limit collagen synthesis by smooth muscle cells, and macrophages, in response to stimulation by T cells, secrete matrix metalloproteinases, which together with collagenase actively degrade the collagen and other extracellular matrix proteins [38], rendering the fibrous cap weak and eventually resulting in plaque rupture.

The rupture of the fibrous cap results in releasing of the prothrombotic lipid content into the lumen: subendothelial collagen, tissue factor, and von Willembrand factor become accessible to circulating components, leading to coagulation and thrombin formation, with platelets activation and aggregation, culminating in acute thrombosis and myocardial infarction.

Inflammation Markers for Prediction of Cardiovascular Risk

Given the pivotal role played by the inflammatory process in the different stages of the atherosclerosis, the analysis of plasma levels of markers of inflammation could help clinicians predicting patient's risk for cardiovascular events and identifying new target for therapeutic intervention [39]. Several candidate markers have been investigated, including primarily inflammatory cytokines, pro-atherogenic enzymes, CAMs, and CRP.

Inflammatory Cytokines

Among the inflammatory cytokines, great interest has been given to IL-6, TNF-α, and CD40/CD40L system.

Among apparently healthy men enrolled in the Physicians' Health Study (PHS), baseline of IL-6 predict indeed future cardiovascular events [40].

The risk of future myocardial infarction increased in parallel with increasing quartile of baseline IL-6 level such that those men in the highest quartile at entry had a relative 2.3 times higher compared with those in the lowest quartile (p=0.005). CRP was the strongest parameter that correlates with IL-6 levels (r=0.43; p<0.001), a data that is consistent with the finding that IL-6 is the main stimulant for both the hepatic and extra-hepatic synthesis of the CRP [26,27]. Moreover, in another study, elevated levels of IL-6 at 48 hours after admission are associated with an adverse in-hospital prognosis among patients with ACS, even without a rise in troponin T [41]. In a study from the secondary prevention Cholesterol and Recurrent Events (CARE) trial, elevation of TNF-α in the stable phase after myocardial infarction were associated with an increased risk of recurrent coronary events [42]. In particular, those with baseline levels over the 95th percentile had a 2.7-fold increase in risk of recurrent events. Furthermore, plasma levels of TNF-α have been shown to correlate with degrees of early atherosclerosis as assessed by carotid ultrasound among healthy middle-aged men and correlate with metabolic and cellular perturbations important for the vascular process, as degrees of alimentary lipaemia, plasma very low density lipoprotein triglyceride, low density lipoprotein (LDL) cholesterol concentrations and peak LDL particle size [43]. Finally, a recent report from the FRagmin during InStability in Coronary artery disease (FRISC) II study group has found that circulating levels of IL-6 are a strong independent marker of increased mortality amongst patients with unstable coronary artery disease and may be useful in directing subsequent care [44]. For examples, randomization to an early invasive strategy led to a 65% relative reduction in 12-month mortality among patients with elevated IL-6 levels. By contrast, among those patients with low IL-6 levels, randomization to an early invasive strategy did not confer any benefit over a non invasive strategy. Moreover, among the patients randomized to the non invasive arm, the risk associated with elevated IL-6 levels was markedly attenuated if they were assigned to therapy with dalteparin rather than placebo [44]. Thus the use of an inflammatory biomarker for risk stratification appears not only to identify patients at high risk for future cardiovascular events, but most importantly to identify individuals who might benefit most from targeted interventional or invasive medical therapy.

As we have already noted earlier in this chapter, the complex CD40 ligand/its receptor CD40 also plays a critical role in the inflammation/atherosclerosis process [16,36]. Interestingly, patients with unstable angina have higher concentrations of functional sCD40L than do patients with stable angina or healthy volunteers, possibly as a result of release from activated platelets or T lymphocytes [45]. To address whether plasma concentrations of sCD40L also have diagnostic or prognostic value among apparently healthy individuals before the onset of acute cardiovascular events, a prospective, nested case-control analysis was performed among participants in the Women's Health Study (WHS), an ongoing primary prevention trial evaluating the efficiency of vitamin E and low-dose aspirin in 28 263 middle-aged American women with no history of cardiovascular disease or cancer [46]. Interestingly, mean concentrations of sCD40L at baseline were significantly higher among 130 participants who subsequently developed myocardial infarction, stroke, or cardiovascular death (cases), compared with 130 age- and smoking-matched women who remained free of cardiovascular disease (controls) during a 4-year follow-up (P=0.02). Women with concentrations above the

95th percentile of the control distribution had a significantly increased relative risk (RR) of developing future cardiovascular events (RR, 3.3; 95% CI, 1.2 to 8.6; P=0.01) that remained after adjustment for usual cardiovascular risk factors [47]. A recent study examining sCD40L in ACS found that elevated sCD40L levels indicated a significantly increased risk of death or non fatal infarction; more interestingly, this risk was reduced significantly by treatment with abciximab, whereas there was no significant treatment effect of abciximab in patients with low levels of soluble CD40 ligand [48]. The authors can then conclude that elevation of soluble CD40 ligand identifies a subgroup of patients at high risk who are likely to benefit from antiplatelet treatment with abciximab. Finally, there are also some evidences that individuals with type 1 or 2 diabetes have higher ($P<0.001$) sCD40L plasma levels compared with age-matched control groups. Troglitazone treatment of type 2 diabetic patients diminishes sCD40L levels, suggesting a novel antiinflammatory mechanism for limiting diabetes-associated arterial disease [49]. Similarly, another study investigated whether the CD40 system is upregulated in patients with moderate hypercholesterolemia and whether it is influenced by therapy with a hydroxymethylglutaryl coenzyme A (HMG-CoA) reductase inhibitor [50]. Patients with moderate hypercholesterolemia showed up regulation of the CD40 system and short-term therapy with cerivastatin, a HMG-CoA reductase inhibitor, significantly down regulated CD40 on monocytes in those patients.

Pro-Atherogenic Enzymes

Other novel inflammatory markers studied as potential predictor of cardiovascular risk include pro-atherogenic enzymes myeloperoxidase (MPO), pregnancy-associated plasma protein A (PAPP-A), and lipoprotein-associated phospholipase A_2 (Lp-PLA_2). MPO is an abundant heme protein stored in primary azurophilic granules of leukocytes and secreted into both the extracellular and the phagolysosomal compartment following phagocyte activation by a variety of agonists [51]. It has been demonstrated to be present in human atherosclerotic lesions [52] and may deplete nitric oxide, leading to endothelial dysfunction, may convert LDL into a high-uptake for of macrophages, leading to the formation of foam cells, and serves as a major enzymatic catalyst of lipid peroxidation at sites of inflammation [53]. In a recent case-control study of patients with and without CAD, increasing levels of both blood-MPO and leukocyte-MPO were significant predictors of the risk for future cardiovascular events [54].

PAPP-A, a zinc-binding matrix metalloproteinase [55], is a specific activator of insulin-like growth factor I, a mediator of atherosclerosis and is probably produced by vascular smooth muscle cells [56]. Because of its matrix metalloproteinase activity, it could be involved in the processing of the plaque's extracellular matrix and weakening of the fibrous cap [2]. This enzyme has been already studied in the setting of the ACS [56]. The authors examined the level of expression of PAPP-A in eight culprit unstable coronary plaques and four stable plaques from eight patients who had died suddenly of cardiac causes. PAPP-A was abundantly expressed in plaque cells and extracellular matrix of ruptured and eroded unstable plaques, but not in stable plaques. They also measured circulating levels of PAPP-A in 17 patients with acute myocardial infarction, 20 with unstable angina, 19 with stable angina, and 13 controls without atherosclerosis. Interestingly, circulating PAPP-A levels were significantly higher in patients with unstable angina or acute myocardial infarction than in patients with stable angina and controls ($P<0.001$). These increased levels may reflect the instability of atherosclerotic plaques. Finally, the role of PAPP-A as a predictor of ischemic cardiac events has been evaluated in a recent study. In cTnI-negative ACS patients, PAPP-A levels ≥2.9 mIU/L were associated with a 4.6-fold higher adjusted risk of adverse outcome compared with patients whose circulating PAPP-A levels were <2.9 mIU/L. In patients with PAPP-A ≥4.5 mIU/L, the risk was even higher [57].

Lp-PLA$_2$, also known as the platelet-activating factor acetylhydrolase, is an enzyme that can hydrolyze oxidized phospholipids to generate lysophosphatidylcholine and oxidized fatty acids, which have proinflammatory properties, is associated primarily with LDL, and enzyme activity is increased in small, dense LDL [58]. In a case–cohort analysis of the West of Scotland Coronary Prevention Study (WOSCOPS), high baseline Lp-PLA2 levels were associated with increased risk for CHD events, even after adjustment for traditional risk factors and hs-CRP [59]. Levels of Lp-PLA$_2$ have also been reported to be significantly elevated in patients with angiographically proven coronary artery disease and appear to serve as an independent predictor of disease status in this population [60]. However, in a case-control analysis from the Women's Health Study, baseline Lp-PLA$_2$ levels were higher in women with subsequent cardiovascular events but were not associated with increased CHD risk after adjustment for traditional risk factors and hs-CRP [61]. Recently, in a prospective, case-cohort study in 12.819 apparently healthy middle-aged men and women in the Atherosclerosis Risk in Communities study (ARIC) [62], the relation between Lp-PLA$_2$, CRP, traditional risk factors, and risk for CHD events over a period of ~ 6 years was examined in a proportional hazards model, stratified by LDL-C. Both Lp-PLA$_2$ and CRP levels were higher in the 608 cases than the 740 noncases. Lp-PLA$_2$ and CRP were also both associated with incident CHD after adjustment for age, sex, and race and, for individuals with LDL-C <130 mg/dL, those with both Lp-PLA$_2$ and CRP levels in the highest tertile were at the greatest risk for a CHD event. Thus, Lp-PLA$_2$ and CRP may be complementary in identifying individuals at high CHD risk who have low LDL-C.

CAMs

Amongst apparently healthy men enrolled in PHS, baseline plasma levels of ICAM-1 were elevated in those who subsequently developed myocardial infarction (MI) compared with those who did not [63]. These data supports the hypothesis that endothelial activation and inflammation occurs early in the atherosclerotic process and that the inflammatory component of the disease is important in influencing future cardiovascular events. The same investigators also recently reported, in a similar prospective epidemiological evaluation of apparently healthy women, that elevation of baseline soluble P-selectin levels was associated with increasing risk of future myocardial infarction, stroke, coronary revascularization and cardiovascular death [64]. This association was again independent of age and persisted after additional control for several lipid and non-lipid cardiovascular risk factors. Similarly, the ARIC study found that baseline levels of ICAM-1 were predictive of both carotid atherosclerosis and future coronary heart disease events and there was also a significant association between levels of sE-selectin and carotid atherosclerosis [65]. Moreover, in the same population from the PHS, baseline plasma levels of ICAM-1 have been found to be associated with systolic blood pressure, mean blood pressure and pulse pressure [66].

In contrast to the strong association between serum levels of sICAM-1 and future cardiovascular events in apparently healthy men and women, the data concerning sVCAM-1 as a marker of future cardiac risk in asymptomatic individuals are less clear. In both ARIC and PHS studies, baseline plasma levels of VCAM-1 were not predictive of future cardiovascular risk amongst apparently healthy individuals [65,67].

However, in a population with previously documented coronary artery disease, baseline plasma levels of both VCAM-1 and ICAM-1 were elevated amongst those who subsequently died because of cardiovascular causes [68]. In adjusted analyses, VCAM-1 was the stronger predictor of risk with an over twofold increased risk of death for the highest compared with the lowest quartile. In the diabetic population, plasma levels of VCAM-1 were found elevated in those patients with symptomatic atherosclerotic vascular disease compared to patients without detectable atherosclerosis, with a positive correlation between VCAM-1 levels and the intima-media thickness of the carotid artery [69]. In another study, using an echographic assessment of the maximum intima-media thickness at the carotid bifurcation in patients with peripheral arterial vascular disease (pAVD), essential hypertension, and healthy controls as a measure of the extent of atherosclerosis, those patients with both pAVD and hypertension revealed higher levels of VCAM-1 compared to those patients only demonstrating hypertension and control [70]. The authors also demonstrated a direct correlation between the maximum intima-media thickness of the carotid artery and the serum levels of VCAM-1; in contrast, levels of ICAM-1 did not correlate with the extent of the intima-media tickness. In another study on 52 patients with pAVD evaluated by angiograms, serum concentration of VCAM-1 correlated with the extent of atherosclerosis according to the Fontaine classes [71].

Finally, there have been a number of reports of elevated levels of cell adhesion molecules in acute coronary syndromes. Shyu et al. reported elevated levels of ICAM-1 in patients with acute coronary syndromes [72]. Ikeda et al. demonstrated elevated levels of P-selectin after an episode of chest pain in patients with unstable angina, but not in those with stable angina or controls [73]. Recently, O'Malley et al. reported elevated levels of ICAM-1 in the majority of patients within hours of the onset of cardiac chest pain [74]. Another group has reported that levels of ICAM-1, VCAM-1 and P-selectin remain elevated throughout the first 72 h after presentation in unstable angina and non Q-wave myocardial infarction, whereas there is a fall in the levels of E-selectin during this time [75]. Moreover, in a prospective study in 20 patients with AMI whose infarct-related coronary artery was successfully recanalized by emergency balloon angioplasty, plasma levels of ICAM-1 at admission, 48 hours, 1 week, and 2 weeks after angioplasty were significantly elevated in patients who had early (3 weeks) restenosis develop compared with those who did not [76]. Acute coronary syndromes are characterized by persistent instability for weeks to months after the resolution of the clinical symptoms resulting in either recurrent episodes of unstable angina, myocardial infarction or death [77]. There is evidence of sustained vascular inflammation following an acute coronary syndrome by the finding of persistent elevation of sICAM-1, sVCAM-1, sE-selectin and sP-selectin for up to 6 months after unstable angina or non Q wave myocardial infarction before a return to levels seen in a stable angina population [78]. These data suggest an association between recurrent ischemic episodes and persistent inflammatory stimuli after an acute coronary event.

CRP

CRP has analytical properties that make it suitable for clinical use, such as a relatively long half-life of 18 hours, lack of circadian variability, plasma levels relatively stable over time, and use on nonfasting samples [79]. Numerous evidences suggest that circulating high-sensitive CRP represents one of the strongest independent predictors of vascular death in a different number of settings [80-82].

Important papers in the early 1990s first showed the association between CRP levels and cardiovascular prognosis amongst patients with unstable coronary syndromes. Liuzzo et al. showed that patients presenting with unstable angina who had elevated plasma levels of CRP (≥3 mg/l) had higher rate of death, AMI, and need for revascularization compared with patients without elevated levels [80-82]. Several following paper have confirmed the prognostic utility of CRP amongst patients with ACS, both in the short- and long-term. The thrombolysis In Myocardial Infarction (TIMI) investigators have described that the increased risk associated with high CRP levels may be evident as early as 14 days after presentation with an ACS [84]. The FRISC investigators found that the risk associated with elevated CRP levels at the time of index event continues to increase for several years [85]. In each of these later studies the predictive value of CRP was independent of, and additive to, that of troponin. Moreover, CRP has been constantly shown to have prognostic value even amongst patients with normal troponin T levels, who have no evidence of myocardial necrosis. Recent data also confirm that CRP is a strong independent predictor of short- and long-term mortality amongst patients with ACS who are treated with very early invasive strategy [86]. Patients with persistently high serum CRP levels might have high probability of occurrence of sub-acute cardiac rupture after AMI [87].

Less consistent are the data for CRP as predictor among patients in the stable phase post-MI. A Norwegian study measured CRP levels in a cohort of 247 patients (193 males and 54 females) who had had their first MI at age < or = 55 (males) or < or = 60 (females) and relative risks for total and cardiac mortality were analyzed. The results suggested that CRP remained a significant predictor for future death in patients with previous premature MI [88]. Moreover, in the CARE study population, the authors studied whether inflammation after MI was a risk factor for recurrent coronary events: interestingly, patients with higher CRP levels were found to be at an increased risk of recurrent cardiovascular events [89]. However, data from the Thrombogenic Factors and Recurrent Coronary Events (THROMBO) study did not confirm these findings. THROMBO was a prospective, multicenter investigation that evaluated the prognostic significance of lipid, inflammatory, and hemostatic factors, measured 2 months after an index MI, for recurrent cardiac events during a subsequent 2-year follow-up period. The results of this study showed that, although univariate analysis revealed a trend toward increasing risk for recurrent coronary events with increasing CRP levels, multivariate analysis revealed that this inflammatory marker was not independent marker for recurrent coronary events after MI [90].

Data in support of a role for CRP for cardiovascular risk prediction amongst apparently healthy individuals are numerous and from large-scale prospective studies. An analysis from the WHS compared the cardiovascular risk associated with baseline levels of CRP with other inflammatory and lipid markers of risk. The cardiovascular events included stroke, nonfatal MI, need for coronary revascularization, and death from coronary heart disease over a mean follow-up of 3 years [80]. Amongst the women who subsequently developed cardiovascular events baseline levels of CRP were significantly elevated at baseline compared with those who did not. Moreover, of all the inflammatory and lipid markers, CRP was the single most powerful predictor of cardiovascular risk. Multivariate analyses, matched for smocking and age, and adjusted for other cardiovascular risk factors, found that only CRP and TC:HDL ratio were independent predictors of future cardiovascular risk. In both men and women, many studies now indicate that the relation between CRP level and future vascular risk is largely independent of cholesterol level, as well as other traditional vascular risk factors [82,91,92]. In a recent study, amongst the participants at the WHS, CRP and LDL cholesterol were recently compared at baseline levels for their ability to predict first MI, ischemic stroke, or coronary revascularization or cardiovascular death [92]. The risk of a first cardiovascular event increased with an increasing quintile for both the markers, but was stronger for CRP than for LDL. In an analysis adjusting for age, smoking status, diabetes, blood pressure, and use of hormone replacement therapy, the relative risks for a future vascular event for increasing quintiles of CRP were also higher compared with those of LDL. Measurement of CRP was found to add substantial prognostic information to the Framingham risk score and to the LDL cholesterol categories of <130 mg/dL, 130 to 160 mg/dL, and >160 mg/dL used in the current National Cholesterol Education Program (NCEP) Adult Treatment Panel (ATP) III guidelines [93]. An increasing CRP quintile remained a significant independent predictor of cardiovascular events after adjustment for all components of the Framingham risk score. In addition to predicting cardiovascular death and MI, CRP is also a robust predictor of stroke [94], as well as the development of peripheral vascular disease [82,95], suggesting that it may have a role in the assessment of global vascular risk [81].

On the basis of these data, the Centers for Disease Control and Prevention and the American Heart Association stated jointly that CRP is an independent marker of risk that may help direct further evaluation and therapy in the primary prevention of cardiovascular disease in patients at intermediate risk [6]. This consensus statement suggested that an increased serum level of CRP in intermediate-risk patients can be used to encourage compliance and health-promoting therapies but should not be used to decide for or against proven therapies for coronary disease.

Conclusions

We are witnessing a tremendous shift in our concept of atherogenesis: atherosclerosis indeed is no longer considered a pure lipid disorder and it has become increasingly clear that a number of mediators of inflammation play a pivotal role in determining atherosclerotic plaque formation and its complications. Numerous emerging evidences suggest that a variety of plasma markers of chronic low-grade vascular wall inflammation may be helpful to predict individuals at high risk for future cardiovascular events. Elevated levels of some adhesion molecules, pro-atherogenic enzymes, cytokines, and particularly CRP have been shown to predict future vascular risk in a variety of clinical settings. CRP has been the most extensively studied, and there is now robust evidences from both primary prevention studies and amongst patients presenting with ACS that elevated levels predict future cardiovascular events. Thus, the addition of screening for these new markers of inflammation to traditional lipid testing has the potential to identify individuals at high risk for future cardiovascular events who may benefit from an aggressive modification of lifestyle and targeted preventive interventions.

REFERENCES

[1] Ross R: Atherosclerosis--an inflammatory disease. *N Engl J Med* 1999, 340:115-126.

[2] Libby P: Inflammation in atherosclerosis. *Nature* 2002, 420:868-874.

[3] Libby P, Ridker PM, Maseri A: Inflammation and atherosclerosis. *Circulation* 2002, 105:1135-1143.

[4] Szmitko PE, Wang CH, Weisel RD, de Almeida JR, Anderson TJ, Verma S: New markers of inflammation and endothelial cell activation: Part I. *Circulation* 2003, 108:1917-1923.

[5] Blake GJ, Ridker PM: Novel clinical markers of vascular wall inflammation. *Circ Res* 2001, 89:763-771.

[6] Pearson TA, Mensah GA, Alexander RW, Anderson JL, Cannon RO, 3rd, Criqui M, Fadl YY, Fortmann SP, Hong Y, Myers GL, et al.: Markers of inflammation and cardiovascular disease: application to clinical and public health practice: A statement for healthcare professionals from the Centers for Disease Control and Prevention and the American Heart Association. *Circulation* 2003, 107:499-511.

[7] Falk E, Shah PK, Fuster V: Coronary plaque disruption. *Circulation* 1995, 92:657-671.

[8] Mann JM, Davies MJ: Vulnerable plaque. Relation of characteristics to degree of stenosis in human coronary arteries. *Circulation* 1996, 94:928-931.

[9] Libby P: Molecular bases of the acute coronary syndromes. *Circulation* 1995, 91:2844-2850.

[10] Tedder TF, Steeber DA, Chen A, Engel P: The selectins: vascular adhesion molecules. *Faseb J* 1995, 9:866-873.

[11] Davies MJ, Gordon JL, Gearing AJ, Pigott R, Woolf N, Katz D, Kyriakopoulos A: The expression of the adhesion molecules ICAM-1, VCAM-1, PECAM, and E-selectin in human atherosclerosis. *J Pathol* 1993, 171:223-229.

[12] Dustin ML, Rothlein R, Bhan AK, Dinarello CA, Springer TA: Induction by IL 1 and interferon-gamma: tissue distribution, biochemistry, and function of a natural adherence molecule (ICAM-1). *J Immunol* 1986, 137:245-254.

[13] Pober JS, Bevilacqua MP, Mendrick DL, Lapierre LA, Fiers W, Gimbrone MA, Jr.: Two distinct monokines, interleukin 1 and tumor necrosis factor, each independently

induce biosynthesis and transient expression of the same antigen on the surface of cultured human vascular endothelial cells. *J Immunol* 1986, 136:1680-1687.

[14] Pober JS, Gimbrone MA, Jr., Lapierre LA, Mendrick DL, Fiers W, Rothlein R, Springer TA: Overlapping patterns of activation of human endothelial cells by interleukin 1, tumor necrosis factor, and immune interferon. *J Immunol* 1986, 137:1893-1896.

[15] Pasceri V, Willerson JT, Yeh ET: Direct proinflammatory effect of C-reactive protein on human endothelial cells. *Circulation* 2000, 102:2165-2168.

[16] Schonbeck U, Libby P: CD40 signaling and plaque instability. *Circ Res* 2001, 89:1092-1103.

[17] Chen M, Masaki T, Sawamura T: LOX-1, the receptor for oxidized low-density lipoprotein identified from endothelial cells: implications in endothelial dysfunction and atherosclerosis. *Pharmacol Ther* 2002, 95:89-100.

[18] Adams DH, Shaw S: Leucocyte-endothelial interactions and regulation of leucocyte migration. *Lancet* 1994, 343:831-836.

[19] Nageh MF, Sandberg ET, Marotti KR, Lin AH, Melchior EP, Bullard DC, Beaudet AL: Deficiency of inflammatory cell adhesion molecules protects against atherosclerosis in mice. *Arterioscler Thromb Vasc Biol* 1997, 17:1517-1520.

[20] Dong ZM, Chapman SM, Brown AA, Frenette PS, Hynes RO, Wagner DD: The combined role of P- and E-selectins in atherosclerosis. *J Clin Invest* 1998, 102:145-152.

[21] Gu L, Okada Y, Clinton SK, Gerard C, Sukhova GK, Libby P, Rollins BJ: Absence of monocyte chemoattractant protein-1 reduces atherosclerosis in low density lipoprotein receptor-deficient mice. *Mol Cell* 1998, 2:275-281.

[22] Qiao JH, Tripathi J, Mishra NK, Cai Y, Tripathi S, Wang XP, Imes S, Fishbein MC, Clinton SK, Libby P, et al.: Role of macrophage colony-stimulating factor in atherosclerosis: studies of osteopetrotic mice. *Am J Pathol* 1997, 150:1687-1699.

[23] Barath P, Fishbein MC, Cao J, Berenson J, Helfant RH, Forrester JS: Detection and localization of tumor necrosis factor in human atheroma. *Am J Cardiol* 1990, 65:297-302.

[24] Sanceau J, Kaisho T, Hirano T, Wietzerbin J: Triggering of the human interleukin-6 gene by interferon-gamma and tumor necrosis factor-alpha in monocytic cells involves cooperation between interferon regulatory factor-1, NF kappa B, and Sp1 transcription factors. *J Biol Chem* 1995, 270:27920-27931.

[25] Rus HG, Vlaicu R, Niculescu F: Interleukin-6 and interleukin-8 protein and gene expression in human arterial atherosclerotic wall. *Atherosclerosis* 1996, 127:263-271.

[26] Heinrich PC, Castell JV, Andus T: Interleukin-6 and the acute phase response. *Biochem J* 1990, 265:621-636.

[27] Calabro P, Willerson JT, Yeh ET: Inflammatory cytokines stimulated C-reactive protein production by human coronary artery smooth muscle cells. *Circulation* 2003, 108:1930-1932.

[28] Verma S, Yeh ET: C-reactive protein and atherothrombosis--beyond a biomarker: an actual partaker of lesion formation. *Am J Physiol Regul Integr Comp Physiol* 2003, 285:R1253-1256; discussion R1257-1258.

[29] Pasceri V, Cheng JS, Willerson JT, Yeh ET, Chang J: Modulation of C-reactive protein-mediated monocyte chemoattractant protein-1 induction in human endothelial cells by anti-atherosclerosis drugs. *Circulation* 2001, 103:2531-2534.

[30] Yeh ET, Anderson HV, Pasceri V, Willerson JT: C-reactive protein: linking inflammation to cardiovascular complications. *Circulation* 2001, 104:974-975.

[31] Verma S, Wang CH, Li SH, Dumont AS, Fedak PW, Badiwala MV, Dhillon B, Weisel RD, Li RK, Mickle DA, et al.: A self-fulfilling prophecy: C-reactive protein attenuates nitric oxide production and inhibits angiogenesis. *Circulation* 2002, 106:913-919.

[32] Verma S, Badiwala MV, Weisel RD, Li SH, Wang CH, Fedak PW, Li RK, Mickle DA: C-reactive protein activates the nuclear factor-kappaB signal transduction pathway in saphenous vein endothelial cells: implications for atherosclerosis and restenosis. *J Thorac Cardiovasc Surg* 2003, 126:1886-1891.

[33] Hattori Y, Matsumura M, Kasai K: Vascular smooth muscle cell activation by C-reactive protein. *Cardiovasc Res* 2003, 58:186-195.

[34] Yeh ET, Willerson JT: Coming of age of C-reactive protein: using inflammation markers in cardiology. *Circulation* 2003, 107:370-371.

[35] Schonbeck U, Libby P: The CD40/CD154 receptor/ligand dyad. *Cell Mol Life Sci* 2001, 58:4-43.

[36] Mach F, Schonbeck U, Bonnefoy JY, Pober JS, Libby P: Activation of monocyte/macrophage functions related to acute atheroma complication by ligation of CD40: induction of collagenase, stromelysin, and tissue factor. *Circulation* 1997, 96:396-399.

[37] Graf D, Muller S, Korthauer U, van Kooten C, Weise C, Kroczek RA: A soluble form of TRAP (CD40 ligand) is rapidly released after T cell activation. *Eur J Immunol* 1995, 25:1749-1754.

[38] Galis ZS, Sukhova GK, Lark MW, Libby P: Increased expression of matrix metalloproteinases and matrix degrading activity in vulnerable regions of human atherosclerotic plaques. *J Clin Invest* 1994, 94:2493-2503.

[39] Ridker PM: Evaluating novel cardiovascular risk factors: can we better predict heart attacks? *Ann Intern Med* 1999, 130:933-937.

[40] Ridker PM, Rifai N, Stampfer MJ, Hennekens CH: Plasma concentration of interleukin-6 and the risk of future myocardial infarction among apparently healthy men. *Circulation* 2000, 101:1767-1772.

[41] Biasucci LM, Liuzzo G, Fantuzzi G, Caligiuri G, Rebuzzi AG, Ginnetti F, Dinarello CA, Maseri A: Increasing levels of interleukin (IL)-1Ra and IL-6 during the first 2 days of hospitalization in unstable angina are associated with increased risk of in-hospital coronary events. *Circulation* 1999, 99:2079-2084.

[42] Ridker PM, Rifai N, Pfeffer M, Sacks F, Lepage S, Braunwald E: Elevation of tumor necrosis factor-alpha and increased risk of recurrent coronary events after myocardial infarction. *Circulation* 2000, 101:2149-2153.

[43] Skoog T, Dichtl W, Boquist S, Skoglund-Andersson C, Karpe F, Tang R, Bond MG, de Faire U, Nilsson J, Eriksson P, et al.: Plasma tumour necrosis factor-alpha and early carotid atherosclerosis in healthy middle-aged men. *Eur Heart J* 2002, 23:376-383.

[44] Lindmark E, Diderholm E, Wallentin L, Siegbahn A: Relationship between interleukin 6 and mortality in patients with unstable coronary artery disease: effects of an early invasive or noninvasive strategy. *Jama* 2001, 286:2107-2113.

[45] Aukrust P, Muller F, Ueland T, Berget T, Aaser E, Brunsvig A, Solum NO, Forfang K, Froland SS, Gullestad L: Enhanced levels of soluble and membrane-bound CD40 ligand in patients with unstable angina. Possible reflection of T lymphocyte and platelet involvement in the pathogenesis of acute coronary syndromes. *Circulation* 1999, 100:614-620.

[46] Rexrode KM, Lee IM, Cook NR, Hennekens CH, Buring JE: Baseline characteristics of participants in the Women's Health Study. *J Womens Health Gend Based Med* 2000, 9:19-27.

[47] Schonbeck U, Varo N, Libby P, Buring J, Ridker PM: Soluble CD40L and cardiovascular risk in women. *Circulation* 2001, 104:2266-2268.

[48] Heeschen C, Dimmeler S, Hamm CW, van den Brand MJ, Boersma E, Zeiher AM, Simoons ML: Soluble CD40 ligand in acute coronary syndromes. *N Engl J Med* 2003, 348:1104-1111.

[49] Varo N, Vicent D, Libby P, Nuzzo R, Calle-Pascual AL, Bernal MR, Fernandez-Cruz A, Veves A, Jarolim P, Varo JJ, et al.: Elevated plasma levels of the atherogenic mediator soluble CD40 ligand in diabetic patients: a novel target of thiazolidinediones. *Circulation* 2003, 107:2664-2669.

[50] Garlichs CD, Kozina S, Fateh-Moghadam S, Handschu R, Tomandl B, Stumpf C, Eskafi S, Raaz D, Schmeisser A, Yilmaz A, et al.: Upregulation of CD40-CD40 ligand (CD154) in patients with acute cerebral ischemia. *Stroke* 2003, 34:1412-1418.

[51] Klebanoff SJ: Myeloperoxidase. *Proc Assoc Am Physicians* 1999, 111:383-389.

[52] Daugherty A, Dunn JL, Rateri DL, Heinecke JW: Myeloperoxidase, a catalyst for lipoprotein oxidation, is expressed in human atherosclerotic lesions. *J Clin Invest* 1994, 94:437-444.

[53] Zhang R, Brennan ML, Shen Z, MacPherson JC, Schmitt D, Molenda CE, Hazen SL: Myeloperoxidase functions as a major enzymatic catalyst for initiation of lipid peroxidation at sites of inflammation. *J Biol Chem* 2002, 277:46116-46122.

[54] Zhang R, Brennan ML, Fu X, Aviles RJ, Pearce GL, Penn MS, Topol EJ, Sprecher DL, Hazen SL: Association between myeloperoxidase levels and risk of coronary artery disease. *Jama* 2001, 286:2136-2142.

[55] Laursen LS, Overgaard MT, Nielsen CG, Boldt HB, Hopmann KH, Conover CA, Sottrup-Jensen L, Giudice LC, Oxvig C: Substrate specificity of the metalloproteinase pregnancy-associated plasma protein-A (PAPP-A) assessed by mutagenesis and analysis of synthetic peptides: substrate residues distant from the scissile bond are critical for proteolysis. *Biochem J* 2002, 367:31-40.

[56] Bayes-Genis A, Conover CA, Overgaard MT, Bailey KR, Christiansen M, Holmes DR, Jr., Virmani R, Oxvig C, Schwartz RS: Pregnancy-associated plasma protein A as a marker of acute coronary syndromes. *N Engl J Med* 2001, 345:1022-1029.

[57] Lund J, Qin QP, Ilva T, Pettersson K, Voipio-Pulkki LM, Porela P, Pulkki K: Circulating pregnancy-associated plasma protein a predicts outcome in patients with

acute coronary syndrome but no troponin I elevation. *Circulation* 2003, 108:1924-1926.

[58] Karabina SA, Liapikos TA, Grekas G, Goudevenos J, Tselepis AD: Distribution of PAF-acetylhydrolase activity in human plasma low-density lipoprotein subfractions. *Biochim Biophys Acta* 1994, 1213:34-38.

[59] Packard CJ, O'Reilly DS, Caslake MJ, McMahon AD, Ford I, Cooney J, Macphee CH, Suckling KE, Krishna M, Wilkinson FE, et al.: Lipoprotein-associated phospholipase A2 as an independent predictor of coronary heart disease. West of Scotland Coronary Prevention Study Group. *N Engl J Med* 2000, 343:1148-1155.

[60] Caslake MJ, Packard CJ, Suckling KE, Holmes SD, Chamberlain P, Macphee CH: Lipoprotein-associated phospholipase A(2), platelet-activating factor acetylhydrolase: a potential new risk factor for coronary artery disease. *Atherosclerosis* 2000, 150:413-419.

[61] Blake GJ, Dada N, Fox JC, Manson JE, Ridker PM: A prospective evaluation of lipoprotein-associated phospholipase A(2) levels and the risk of future cardiovascular events in women. *J Am Coll Cardiol* 2001, 38:1302-1306.

[62] Ballantyne CM, Hoogeveen RC, Bang H, Coresh J, Folsom AR, Heiss G, Sharrett AR: Lipoprotein-Associated Phospholipase A2, High-Sensitivity C-Reactive Protein, and Risk for Incident Coronary Heart Disease in Middle-Aged Men and Women in the Atherosclerosis Risk in Communities (ARIC) Study. *Circulation* 2004.

[63] Ridker PM, Hennekens CH, Roitman-Johnson B, Stampfer MJ, Allen J: Plasma concentration of soluble intercellular adhesion molecule 1 and risks of future myocardial infarction in apparently healthy men. *Lancet* 1998, 351:88-92.

[64] Ridker PM, Buring JE, Rifai N: Soluble P-selectin and the risk of future cardiovascular events. *Circulation* 2001, 103:491-495.

[65] Hwang SJ, Ballantyne CM, Sharrett AR, Smith LC, Davis CE, Gotto AM, Jr., Boerwinkle E: Circulating adhesion molecules VCAM-1, ICAM-1, and E-selectin in carotid atherosclerosis and incident coronary heart disease cases: the Atherosclerosis Risk In Communities (ARIC) study. *Circulation* 1997, 96:4219-4225.

[66] Chae CU, Lee RT, Rifai N, Ridker PM: Blood pressure and inflammation in apparently healthy men. *Hypertension* 2001, 38:399-403.

[67] de Lemos JA, Hennekens CH, Ridker PM: Plasma concentration of soluble vascular cell adhesion molecule-1 and subsequent cardiovascular risk. *J Am Coll Cardiol* 2000, 36:423-426.

[68] Blankenberg S, Rupprecht HJ, Bickel C, Peetz D, Hafner G, Tiret L, Meyer J: Circulating cell adhesion molecules and death in patients with coronary artery disease. *Circulation* 2001, 104:1336-1342.

[69] Otsuki M, Hashimoto K, Morimoto Y, Kishimoto T, Kasayama S: Circulating vascular cell adhesion molecule-1 (VCAM-1) in atherosclerotic NIDDM patients. *Diabetes* 1997, 46:2096-2101.

[70] De Caterina R, Basta G, Lazzerini G, Dell'Omo G, Petrucci R, Morale M, Carmassi F, Pedrinelli R: Soluble vascular cell adhesion molecule-1 as a biohumoral correlate of atherosclerosis. *Arterioscler Thromb Vasc Biol* 1997, 17:2646-2654.

[71] Peter K, Nawroth P, Conradt C, Nordt T, Weiss T, Boehme M, Wunsch A, Allenberg J, Kubler W, Bode C: Circulating vascular cell adhesion molecule-1 correlates with the extent of human atherosclerosis in contrast to circulating intercellular adhesion molecule-1, E-selectin, P-selectin, and thrombomodulin. *Arterioscler Thromb Vasc Biol* 1997, 17:505-512.

[72] Shyu KG, Chang H, Lin CC, Kuan P: Circulating intercellular adhesion molecule-1 and E-selectin in patients with acute coronary syndrome. *Chest* 1996, 109:1627-1630.

[73] Ikeda H, Takajo Y, Ichiki K, Ueno T, Maki S, Noda T, Sugi K, Imaizumi T: Increased soluble form of P-selectin in patients with unstable angina. *Circulation* 1995, 92:1693-1696.

[74] O'Malley T, Ludlam CA, Riemermsa RA, Fox KA: Early increase in levels of soluble inter-cellular adhesion molecule-1 (sICAM-1); potential risk factor for the acute coronary syndromes. *Eur Heart J* 2001, 22:1226-1234.

[75] Mulvihill N, Foley JB, Ghaisas N, Murphy R, Crean P, Walsh M: Early temporal expression of soluble cellular adhesion molecules in patients with unstable angina and subendocardial myocardial infarction. *Am J Cardiol* 1999, 83:1265-1267, A1269.

[76] Kamijikkoku S, Murohara T, Tayama S, Matsuyama K, Honda T, Ando M, Hayasaki K: Acute myocardial infarction and increased soluble intercellular adhesion molecule-1: a marker of vascular inflammation and a risk of early restenosis? *Am Heart J* 1998, 136:231-236.

[77] Mulcahy R, Daly L, Graham I, Hickey N, O'Donoghue S, Owens A, Ruane P, Tobin G: Unstable angina: natural history and determinants of prognosis. *Am J Cardiol* 1981, 48:525-528.

[78] Mulvihill NT, Foley JB, Murphy R, Crean P, Walsh M: Evidence of prolonged inflammation in unstable angina and non-Q wave myocardial infarction. *J Am Coll Cardiol* 2000, 36:1210-1216.

[79] Yeh ET, Palusinski RP: C-reactive protein: the pawn has been promoted to queen. *Curr Atheroscler Rep* 2003, 5:101-105.

[80] Ridker PM, Hennekens CH, Buring JE, Rifai N: C-reactive protein and other markers of inflammation in the prediction of cardiovascular disease in women. *N Engl J Med* 2000, 342:836-843.

[81] Ridker PM: High-sensitivity C-reactive protein: potential adjunct for global risk assessment in the primary prevention of cardiovascular disease. *Circulation* 2001, 103:1813-1818.

[82] Ridker PM, Stampfer MJ, Rifai N: Novel risk factors for systemic atherosclerosis: a comparison of C-reactive protein, fibrinogen, homocysteine, lipoprotein(a), and standard cholesterol screening as predictors of peripheral arterial disease. *Jama* 2001, 285:2481-2485.

[83] Liuzzo G, Biasucci LM, Gallimore JR, Grillo RL, Rebuzzi AG, Pepys MB, Maseri A: The prognostic value of C-reactive protein and serum amyloid a protein in severe unstable angina. *N Engl J Med* 1994, 331:417-424.

[84] Morrow DA, Rifai N, Antman EM, Weiner DL, McCabe CH, Cannon CP, Braunwald E: C-reactive protein is a potent predictor of mortality independently of and in

combination with troponin T in acute coronary syndromes: a TIMI 11A substudy. Thrombolysis in Myocardial Infarction. *J Am Coll Cardiol* 1998, 31:1460-1465.

[85] Lindahl B, Toss H, Siegbahn A, Venge P, Wallentin L: Markers of myocardial damage and inflammation in relation to long-term mortality in unstable coronary artery disease. FRISC Study Group. Fragmin during Instability in Coronary Artery Disease. *N Engl J Med* 2000, 343:1139-1147.

[86] Mueller C, Buettner HJ, Hodgson JM, Marsch S, Perruchoud AP, Roskamm H, Neumann FJ: Inflammation and long-term mortality after non-ST elevation acute coronary syndrome treated with a very early invasive strategy in 1042 consecutive patients. *Circulation* 2002, 105:1412-1415.

[87] Ueda S, Ikeda U, Yamamoto K, Takahashi M, Nishinaga M, Nago N, Shimada K: C-reactive protein as a predictor of cardiac rupture after acute myocardial infarction. *Am Heart J* 1996, 131:857-860.

[88] Retterstol L, Eikvar L, Bohn M, Bakken A, Erikssen J, Berg K: C-reactive protein predicts death in patients with previous premature myocardial infarction--a 10 year follow-up study. *Atherosclerosis* 2002, 160:433-440.

[89] Ridker PM, Rifai N, Pfeffer MA, Sacks FM, Moye LA, Goldman S, Flaker GC, Braunwald E: Inflammation, pravastatin, and the risk of coronary events after myocardial infarction in patients with average cholesterol levels. Cholesterol and Recurrent Events (CARE) Investigators. *Circulation* 1998, 98:839-844.

[90] Harb TS, Zareba W, Moss AJ, Ridker PM, Marder VJ, Rifai N, Miller Watelet LF, Arora R, Brown MW, Case RB, et al.: Association of C-reactive protein and serum amyloid A with recurrent coronary events in stable patients after healing of acute myocardial infarction. *Am J Cardiol* 2002, 89:216-221.

[91] Ridker PM, Cushman M, Stampfer MJ, Tracy RP, Hennekens CH: Inflammation, aspirin, and the risk of cardiovascular disease in apparently healthy men. *N Engl J Med* 1997, 336:973-979.

[92] Ridker PM, Rifai N, Rose L, Buring JE, Cook NR: Comparison of C-reactive protein and low-density lipoprotein cholesterol levels in the prediction of first cardiovascular events. *N Engl J Med* 2002, 347:1557-1565.

[93] Executive Summary of The Third Report of The National Cholesterol Education Program (NCEP) Expert Panel on Detection, Evaluation, And Treatment of High Blood Cholesterol In Adults (Adult Treatment Panel III). *Jama* 2001, 285:2486-2497.

[94] Rost NS, Wolf PA, Kase CS, Kelly-Hayes M, Silbershatz H, Massaro JM, D'Agostino RB, Franzblau C, Wilson PW: Plasma concentration of C-reactive protein and risk of ischemic stroke and transient ischemic attack: the Framingham study. *Stroke* 2001, 32:2575-2579.

[95] Ridker PM, Cushman M, Stampfer MJ, Tracy RP, Hennekens CH: Plasma concentration of C-reactive protein and risk of developing peripheral vascular disease. *Circulation* 1998, 97:425-428.

In: Current Topics in Atherosclerosis Research
Editor: Yong J. Geng, pp. 67-79
ISBN 1-59454-428-X

Chapter IV

NITRIC OXIDE BIOLOGY AND ATHEROSCLEROSIS

Ka Bian* and Ferid Murad*

Department of Integrative Biology and Pharmacology School of Medicine,
Institute of Molecular Medicine
University of Texas, Health Science Center at Houston

ABSTRACT

Growing evidence indicates that atherosclerosis is a chronic inflammatory process. The arterial wall has been considered as a major source of reactive species (RS) that include nitric oxide ($^{\bullet}NO$), superoxide ($O_2^{\bullet -}$) and hydrogen peroxide (H_2O_2). Physiological levels of reactive species actively participate in vascular biological activity as second messengers and reagents. But, the excess generation of reactive species contributes to the initiation and progression of vascular injury, such as atherosclerosis. Recognizing the central role of oxidation in the pathogenesis of atherosclerosis has led to intense interests in the potential role of NO_2-Tyr formation in the atherosclerotic plaque. The formation of nitrated proteins and their identification, the functional consequences of protein nitration, and the metabolism of nitrated proteins are all of interest, yet they are unresolved topics of nitric oxide research. The common feature of all putative mechanisms of protein nitration is the direct or indirect dependence of H_2O_2. The H_2O_2 molecule is an intracellular messenger that regulates different signaling pathways through stimulation of tyrosine phosphorylation and is deeply involved in atherosclerosis and vascular remodeling. Our recent studies have indicated that H_2O_2 is fundamentally important in protein oxidation that forms the basis for protein nitration. However, molecular mechanism(s) underlying the role of H_2O_2 in balancing either nitration or

---

* Correspondence concerning this article should be addressed to Drs Ka Bian and Ferid Murad, Department of Integrated Biology and Pharmacology, and the Institute of Molecular Medicine, University of Texas Health Science Center at Houston, TX77030. Email Addresses: ka.bian@uth.tmc.edu, ferid.murad@uth.tmc.edu.

phosphorylation of tyrosine residues require further examination. The proper control of reactive species may be important in the prevention and treatment of atherosclerosis.

Keywords: Nitric Oxide Biology, Signal Transduction, Nitrotyrosine, Free Radicals, Atherosclerosis.

Introduction

The blood vessel bed has to face enormous stress such as blood stream shear force and constantly generated reactive oxygen and nitrogen species. A healthy vascular homeostasis is heavily dependent on the integrity of the endothelium that is a dynamic autocrine and paracrine organ with vasodilator, anti-inflammatory, and antithrombotic properties [1]. Dysfunction of the endothelial cells and loss of endothelium-derived nitric oxide ($^{\bullet}NO$) are major critical factors in the pathogenesis of vascular diseases including atherosclerosis.

A substantial knowledge of the NO signaling pathway has been gained during the past two decades. In 1977, Murad has reported that "nitrovasodilators" such as nitroglycerin and nitroprusside exerted smooth muscle dilation via generation of NO that activated soluble guanylyl cyclase and increased concentration of cGMP in the tissues [2]. Nitric oxide is function as a messenger was proposed first the time. Furchgott [3] further described an endothelium-derived vasodilator factor that has been identified as nitric oxide. In addition to its discovery as a vasodilator, NO mediates several protective functions of the endothelium by inhibiting:

1) neutrophil activation and adhesion; 2) platelet adhesion and aggregation; 3) vascular smooth muscle proliferation; 4) expression of pro-inflammatory cytokines. Thus, a healthy endothelium with normal generation of NO acts to prevent atherosclerosis development and its complications.

In contrast to the effect of physiological concentrations of NO, large amounts of NO can be toxic and pro-inflammatory. For example, $^{\bullet}NO$ reacts with $O_2^{\bullet -}$ to form peroxynitrite ($ONOO^-$) that can further form its acid form, peroxynitrous acid (ONOOH), a very unstable and reactive oxidizing species. Involvement of $ONOO^-$ in inflammatory diseases has been determined by detection of nitrotyrosine (NO_2-Tyr) formation in various inflamed tissues [4,5]. Nitrite (NO_2^-) is another major oxidation product derived from NO, and can be oxidized by peroxidase to form a reactive nitrogen intermediate(s) such as nitrogen dioxide that is capable of nitrating tyrosine. MPO and other peroxidase are also able to use halides and pseudohalides as co-substrates to generate the reactive intermediate hypochlorous acid, which further forms nitryl chloride that results in formation of NO2-Tyr [6]. Thus, it is likely that multiple pathways participate in tyrosine nitration which we will further describe in this chapter.

Protein Nitration and Atherosclerosis

Protein tyrosine nitration is a post-translational modification of proteins. Nitrated proteins are continuously produced in cells by reactive oxygen and nitrogen species even under normal physiological conditions [5]. During periods of inflammation, protein nitration is significantly increased and may become a threat to cell survival. It is well accepted that protein tyrosine nitration could be a biomarker to evaluate the extent and perhaps cause of tissue damage. In addition, the nitration of proteins has been postulated to alter a protein's conformation and structure, catalytic activity, and/or susceptibility to protease digestion [7]. It has been shown that tyrosine nitration can diminish a protein's effectiveness as a substrate for tyrosine kinases [8]. Furthermore, nitrated proteins may exacerbate the pathogenic process and play a role in the connection between inflammation and complications.

Evidence is increasing that inflammatory mechanisms are important participants in the pathophysiology of atherosclerosis [9]. The signs of inflammation have been observed at the earliest identifiable lesion (fatty streak) and the endothelial dysfunction that results from the initial insult further promotes the inflammatory reaction such as increased synthesis of vasoactive molecules, cytokines and procoagulant factors. The adhesiveness of the endothelium to leukocytes and platelets and the heavy infiltration of cellular components (such as monocytes, macrophages and T lymphocytes) within the arterial wall is one of the major inflammatory pathologic changes. The inflammatory response eventually forms foam cells with intimal thickening, plaque formation, and vessel narrowing. Persistent inflammation creates the best condition for reactive species production and oxidative and nitrative stress in atherosclerotic lesions which is of fundamental importance in the development of protein nitration.

As a major molecular marker of oxidative events, association of NO_2-Tyr levels with cardiovascular disease has been extensively studied [7] and substantive nitrated protein tyrosines has been detected in human atherosclerosis by immunohistochemistry [10] with both polyclonal and monoclonal antibodies. Protein nitration was pronounced in and around foamy macrophages within the atheroma deposits. Nitration was also observed in early subintimal fatty streaks. However, Evans P et al's study [11] has questioned whether human atherosclerotic lesions contain NO_2-Tyr. Their studies of normal human aortic intima and atherosclerotic lesions at various stages of development failed to reveal presence of NO_2-Tyr except in a very few specimens of both normal and diseased tissues. The techniques this group has used included HPLC with photodiode array detection and Western blotting which were able to identify NO_2-Tyr after chemical nitration. It should be noted that HPLC detecting of NO_2-Tyr involves enzymatic hydrolysis of protein and other procedures. A number of factors may inflence the accuracy of the measurement. Sample hydrolysis vials made of different materials may also affact the outcomes of NO_2-Tyr measurement. It was found that the 3-nitro- and 3-amino-derivatives of tyrosine were not stable to hydrolysis in glass, and the remedy to this problem was the use of polypropylene Eppendorf tubes [12]. In addition, the protection of samples from damage during hydrolysis is another issue that should be considered. Several experiments have been performed in order to find a highly sensitive and specific analytical method for quantifying free and protein-bound 3-NO_2-Tyr. Using reverse-phase HPLC with the samples of atherosclerotic vessels obtained from the patients who underwent either coronary artery or peripheric artery bypass surgery, Sucu et al (Sucu et al. 2003) reported a significant elevation of NO_2-Tyr levels in atherosclerotic vessels (46.6 +/- 23.3 nmol/mg protein, n = 15; $p < 0.001$) in comparison to that in control vessels (15.8 +/- 2.5 nmol/mg protein, n = 10). Morton et al [12] have employed GLC-MS measuring of NO_2-Tyr formation in advanced human carotid plaque. Despite the existence of tyrosine nitration, their study indicated that the frequency of nitration was 92+/-15 micro mol/mol of tyrosine (0.01%) which accounted for approx. 3% of the tyrosine modifications measured. Thus, the contribution of nitration to the total pool of modified tyrosine is relative small. However, the possibility of metabolic processes or chemical agents modifying 3-NO_2-Tyr to secondary oxidation products remains an alternative explanation for the low levels demonstrated in this study.

In atherosclerosis, the presence of a large numbers of foam cells in the intima may enhance inflammatory reactions by producing a high concentration of pro-infammatory cytokines and growth factors within localized lesion areas. The inflammation can be further propagated by endothelial cells, other cellular elements of the vessel wall, as well as the atherosclerotic plaque itself, which results in the production of adhesive molecules, cytokines and growth factors that amplify the pathologic process. It was demonstrated [14] that extracellular superoxide dismutase (EC-SOD) and inducible nitric oxide synthase (iNOS) are highly expressed in macrophages in human atherosclerotic lesions which colocalization with epitopes characteristic of oxidized LDL and nitrated proteins. In addition, widely expressed cyclooxygenase-2 is also reported in atherosclerotic lesions where iNOS and NO_2-Tyr were detected [15], thus, the formation of NO_2-Tyr further indicated a major role of inflammation in the development of atherosclerotic lesions.

It is well known that oxidized low density lipoprotein (LDL) is of central importance in triggering atherosclerosis. Leeuwenburgh et al [16] has proposed that reactive nitrogen intermediates promote low density lipoprotein oxidation in human atherosclerotic intima. By using LDL samples isolated from human atherosclerotic tissue during autopsy, the group demonstrated that there was a striking 90-fold increase in the level of protein-bound 3-NO_2-Tyr in lesion LDL compared with that in circulating LDL.

To further correlate protein nitration with defective vascular function of atherosclerotic lesions, Zou et al [17] studied selective nitration of prostacyclin synthase in atherosclerotic bovine coronary arteries. Prostacyclin synthase (PCS) is an enzyme with antithrombotic, antiproliferative, and dilatory functions in the normal vasculature. During the early stage of atherosclerotic lesions (focal intimal thickenings), PCS is the major detectable nitrated protein that can be further degraded into two smaller products with molecular mass of 30 and 46 kd. Acompanying PCS nitration, agonist (acetylcholine, angiotensin II)-induced prostacyclin formation was decreased in atherosclerotic vessels compared with normal tissue, whereas PGE2 formation was increased and cyclooxygenase activity remained unchanged. Direct measurement of enzymatic activity further confirmed the selective loss of PCS activity. As the consequence, the early atherosclerotic vessels demonstrated an attenuated vasodilation. This functional impairment was completely reversed by coincubation with an antagonist of the thromboxane/PGH2 receptor but not by a thromboxane synthase inhibitor. This study suggests that protein nitration of PCS reduces its enzymic activity in atherosclerotic arteries which prevents the rapid use of PGH2. The accumulated PGH2 acts as an agonist on the vasoconstrictive thromboxane receptor.

Formation of nitrated protein in atherosclerosis has also been linked to associated thrombotic complications. Bar-Shavit et al [18] have reported that nitration of tyrosine residues of thrombin promoted endothelial cell adhesion while native thrombin exhibited a relative low cell attachment activity. Recently, Vadseth et al [19] has further defined that post translational modification of fibrinogen by reactive nitrogen species promoted pro-thrombotic state. Their research demonstrated that exposure of fibrinogen to nitrating oxidants significantly accelerates clot formation and factor XIII cross-linking, whereas exposure of fibrinogen to non-nitrating oxidants decreas clot formation. Clots formed with fibrinogen exposed to nitrating oxidants are composed of large bundles made from twisted thin fibrin fibers with increased permeation and a decrease in storage modulus G value, suggesting that these clots could be easily deformed by mechanical stresses. In contrast, clots formed with fibrinogen exposed to non-nitrating oxidants showed decreased permeation with normal architecture. Fibrinogen modified by exposure to physiologic nitration systems demonstrated no difference in the rate of plasmin-induced clot lysis, platelet aggregation or binding. Therefore, the study concludes that increased levels of fibrinogen nitration may lead to a pro-thrombotic state via acceleration in formation of fibrin clots.

Nonenzymatic (Transition Metal) Pathway of Protein Tyrosine Nitration

Vertebrates constantly generate reactive oxygen species (ROS), which include superoxide anion ($O_2^{\bullet -}$), hydroxyl radicals ($^{\bullet}OH$) and hydrogen peroxide (H_2O_2) as a consequence of aerobic metabolism. The overproduced ROS have detrimental effects on cellular function in large part through the oxidation of proteins. The discovery of nitric oxide [20] focused attention on reactive nitrogen species (RNS), which includes $^{\bullet}NO$ (nitrogen monoxide) that can under go interconversion to form NO+ (nitrosonium), and NO^- (nitroxyl anion). $^{\bullet}NO$ reacts with $O_2^{\bullet -}$ to form peroxynitrite ($ONOO^-$) that can further form peroxynitrous acid (ONOOH), a very unstable and reactive oxidizing species. Involvement of ONOO is the most widely studied mechanism of protein nitration [21], and the formation of NO_2-Tyr has been detected in various pathological conditions including atherosclerosis that has been reviewed above.

Nevertheless, substantial evidence has emerged which revealed a very close association between the formation of NO_2-Tyr and the presence of activated granulocytes containing peroxidases, such as myeloperoxidase (MPO) [22,23,24]. MPO-generated oxidants enhance selective cleavage of plasmalogens, a predominant membrane constituent in many cells of the cardiovascular system, and result in the release of both α-chloro fatty aldehyde species, such as 2-chlorohexadecanal that may act as a phagocyte chemoattractant, and unsaturated lysophosphatidylcholine, an as-yet unrecognized proatherogenic molecule because it elicits increased surface expression of P-selectin on human coronary [25]. MPO-generated reactive species participate in the induction of foam cell formation, endothelial dysfunction, and development of vulnerable plaque. Thus, a role for MPO as a mediator of atherosclerosis has received considerable attention. Two radical intermediates have been proposed to play a key role in peroxidase catalyzed nitration of phenolic rings [8]. First, on addition of H_2O_2, MPO (ground state with ferric form) can be oxidized to form compound I (ferryl cation radical) that is readily reduced to form hypochlorous acid (HOCl) in the presence of physiological concentrations of chloride. The reaction could then proceed by Cl transfer from HOCl to nitrite (NO_2^-) to generate nitryl chloride (NO_2Cl) as a reaction intermediate. The second radical intermediate is nitrogen dioxide ($NO_2^•$), which can be generated via either compound I- or II-catalyzed oxidation of NO_2^-. In addition, it has been suggested that physiological concentrations of NO_2^- can be oxidized to $^•NO_2$ by the Fenton reaction [26], a Fe^{2+}-dependent reaction during which decomposition of H_2O_2 forms hydroxyl radical ($^•OH$) that oxidizes NO_2^- to $NO_2^•$.

Peroxidases are enzymes that use H_2O_2 to oxidize substrates. In addition to MPO, the family of human peroxidases includes eosinophil peroxidase, lactoperoxidase, thyroid peroxidase, and intestinal peroxidase [27], all of which share heme-containing homology and can catalyze oxidative reactions. In addition, due to structural similarities, several hemoproteins such as cytochrome P450 isoenzymes, prostaglandin endoperoxide synthase (prostaglandin H synthase), cytochrome c, and hemoglobin are expected to act more or less as an oxidant [26]. The biological role of heme has been reviewed extensively [28,29], and the heme molecule has been shown to promote most biological oxidation processes involved in oxygen transport, mitochondrial respiration, drug metabolism, steroid biosynthesis, cellular antioxidant defenses, and signal transduction processes [30,31]. The presence of heme and peroxides may modulate vascular cell survival and oxidative stress adaptation, thus providing a possible mechanism for the evolution of atherosclerotic lesions [32]. Heme is a complex of protoporphyrin IX with iron that is pentacoordinated and in the high-spin Fe (III) oxidation state. Iron has the capacity to accept and donate electrons readily and to interconvert between ferric (Fe^{3+}) and ferrous (Fe^{2+}), which makes it a useful component of hemoproteins or metalloproteins. However, as a transition metal, iron is able to reduce (active) molecular oxygen and to catalyze the conversion of superoxide and hydrogen peroxide to free radical species. Thus, the iron-containing structure of heme is an oxidant in several model systems where the prooxidant effects of free iron, heme, and hemoprotein may be attributed to the formation of free radical species and hypervalent states of the heme iron that attack cellular components. Recently, we have tested the hypothesis that both free heme and iron play a key role in NO_2-Tyr formation and demonstrated that isolated heme and free metals are capable of tyrosine nitration in the presence of hydrogen peroxide and nitrite. Our studies [33] have made several important discussions on the mechanisms underlying the hemin/iron catalyzed nitration:

Heme-Catalyzed Protein Nitration

Incubation of BSA with various combinations of heme, nitrite and H2O2 in phosphate buffer at physiological pH for 30 min can result in BSA nitration. All components of the heme/ NO_2^-/H_2O_2 system are critical for NO_2-Tyr formation. To further confirm the requirements of the reaction, we used glucose/glucose oxidase (10 mM/100 units) to generate the H_2O_2 (27) which also induced BSA NO_2-Tyr formation. Our experiment indicated that the heme (25 μM) catalyzed BSA tyrosine nitration is comparable with the nitration induced by 5 mM peroxynitrite.

The Role of H_2O_2

To further elucidate the biochemical basis of protein nitration by heme/ NO_2^-/H_2O_2 system, we investigated the carbonyl formation and NO_2-Tyr formation as markers of protein oxidation and nitration respectively and revealed that nitration and oxidation are two distinguishable processes. By dissecting of those two reactions, we were able to conclude that despite the fundamental important role of H_2O_2 in heme (or Fe) catalyzed nitration, high concentrations of H_2O_2 markedly reduced the level of protein nitration by hemin while exerting less effect on BSA oxidation. We also stated that a decreased extent of nitration may reflect the degradation of heme by higher concentrations of H_2O_2 since without the heme structure, iron catalyzed BSA nitration was positively correlated with the increased concentration of H_2O_2.

The Role of Nitrite

Nitrite has been recognized as one of the key oxidation products of NO. NO_2^- is a small molecule with high affinity for the heme center in peroxidase, which has been reported to enhance the oxidizing capacity of peroxidase/H2O2 (28). In the presence of heme and H2O2, we observed a strong NO_2^-.concentration-dependent nitration ($r = 0.98$) of BSA. In contrast, carbonyl formation showed no relationship ($r = 0$) with nitrite concentration.

Explore the Mechanism Responsible for the Heme (iron)-Mediated Nitration

Heme-containing enzymes are involved in both reduction and activation of oxygen. In the heme molecule, five of the coordination sites of iron are occupied by intrinsic ligands, and the sixth is able to bind O_2 or other extrinsic ligands. The strong and symmetrical coordination of the axial ligands enhances the interaction between O_2 and iron-porphyrin and results in the formation of $O_2^{\bullet-}$ by reduction of O_2 [34]. As we know, superoxide dismutase (SOD) interferes with the reactive oxygen species and reactive nitrogen species generating system by converting $O_2^{\bullet-}$ into H_2O_2. This will reduce the formation of $ONOO^-$ but increase the concentration of H_2O_2, which, in the presence of transition metals such as iron can generate a strong oxidant, hydroxyl radical ($^{\bullet}OH$), via the Fenton reaction. However, another heme-containing enzyme catalase can degrade H_2O_2 to water and oxygen thus inhibiting $^{\bullet}OH$ formation. To evaluate the effect of SOD and catalase on protein nitration, we used heme as well as MPO to catalyze BSA NO_2-Tyr formation. Treatment with SOD had no significant effect on BSA nitration. In contrast, the application of catalase abolished both heme and

MPO-induced protein tyrosine nitration. Thus, the above results further confirmed the requirement for H_2O_2 in protein nitration by the heme/$O_2^{\bullet-}$/H_2O_2 system. Although the inhibitory effect of catalase on heme- or Fe-catalyzed nitration may suggest the involvement of the Fenton reaction as suggested by Thomas *et al.* [35], our data have revealed that a potent hydroxyl radical scavenger, mannitol together with EtOH, had no effect on Fe-catalyzed BSA tyrosine nitration. Thus, heme/iron-mediated protein nitration does not depend on the formation of hydroxyl radical. In addition, Fenton reaction effectively produces hydroxyl radical in several seconds; however, our study showed that a 16-h incubation is needed for iron to induce BSA nitration. Thus, the inefficiency of the iron/H_2O_2/NO_2^-/system in protein nitration casts further doubt on the role of hydroxyl radical in iron-catalyzed tyrosine nitration.

Formation of a Fe(IV) Hypervalent Compound may be Essential for Heme(Fe) Catalyzed Nitration

The release of iron in an oxidative manner from heme-containing proteins has received consideration recently [36]. As a transition element, iron is able to exist in several oxidative states in response to different liganding environments [37]. Therefore, we tested whether iron or chelated iron has a catalytic effect on tyrosine nitration. According to our study, both ferrous and ferric ions are capable of catalyzing the nitration of BSA at tyrosine residues when incubated with BSA in the presence of NO_2^- and H_2O_2. To study the mechanism, cyanide (CN^-) and EDTA were used as chelators when addition of iron first into the BSA containing mixture, followed by adding of CN^- or EDTA, significant BSA nitration, was detected. Nitration also was detected if the iron was mixed with EDTA before adding to the BSA-containing reaction buffer. However, if the iron was first mixed with cyanide then added to the BSA-containing buffer, no protein nitration was observed. Of interest, addition of EDTA partly reversed the inhibited nitration by the premixture of iron with cyanide, whereas the addition of cyanide into an iron-EDTA mixture markedly enhanced NO_2-Tyr formation. Thus, the sequential addition of iron and cyanide and the mixture of iron and cyanide first before application into the BSA-containing buffer created completely opposite results in terms of protein nitration. As a potent iron-chelating agent, CN^- can occupy all of the binding sites of iron in a 6:1 ratio and completely block the catalytic effect of iron on BSA nitration. Incomplete binding characteristics of either EDTA or BSA [38] are useful for iron to form its redox status [Fe(IV)] [37] that may further be stabilized by addition of CN^-. Summarizing current information, the catalytic effect of heme or chelated iron on the BSA tyrosine nitration could be described by following reaction (Eqs. 1-4):

$$H - He - Fe(III) + H_2O_2 \rightarrow He^{\bullet} - Fe(IV) - OH^- + H_2O \quad (1)$$

$$He^{\bullet} - Fe(IV) - OH^- + NO_2^- + H^+ \rightarrow H - He - Fe(IV) - OH^- + {}^{\bullet}NO_2 \quad (2)$$

$$He^{\bullet} - Fe(IV) - OH^- + Tyr - H \rightarrow H - He - Fe(IV) - OH^- + Tyr^{\bullet} \quad (3)$$

$$Tyr^{\bullet} + {}^{\bullet}NO_2 \rightarrow NO_2 - Tyr \quad (4)$$

Briefly, hemin or chelated iron reacts with H_2O_2 to form the ferryl π-cation radical complex, which then oxidizes both nitrite and tyrosine to form nitric dioxide radical (${}^{\bullet}NO_2$) and tyrosine radical ($Tyr^{\bullet}$), respectively. These nitrating species nitrate tyrosyl residues in proteins to form NO_2-Tyr.

Cardiovascular System, A Major Target for Protein Nitration:

The average adult human body contains ≈3-4 g of iron, and 65% of it is bound to hemoglobin. Ten percent is a constituent of myoglobin, cytochromes, and iron-containing enzymes, and the rest is bound to the iron storage proteins [39]. The higher contents of iron (heme) in certain tissues such as heart and vascular smooth muscle cells could serve as a biological base for iron toxicity on free radical-mediated tissue damage, including formation of nitrotyrosine. The first evidence [40] that muscle contraction can be altered by nitration of key proteins is suggested by the study of skeletal muscle sarcoplasmic-reticulum (SR) Ca^{2+}-ATPase isoforms 2 (SERCA2a), which suggests that tyrosine nitration may affect Ca^{2+}-ATPase activity. In light of the possibility that a high concentration of heme may facilitate protein nitration, we compared NO_2-Tyr formation in tissue homogenates from various organs. In the presence of heme, H_2O_2 and NO_2^-, considerable protein nitration was observed in homogenates of heart and skeleton muscle but not in the brain, liver, and kidney. Increasing the exogenous heme concentration, however, promoted nitration in the brain, liver, and kidney. To further elucidate the role of endogenous heme in NO_2-Tyr formation, we compared protein nitration in homogenates of heart under conditions of with or without exogenous heme. A significant protein nitration could be induced by application of NO_2^- and H_2O_2 alone into the heart homogenate, and the addition of exogenous heme did not further increase the level of NO_2-Tyr formation. Thus, hemoprotein rich tissues such as cardiac muscle are vulnerable to protein nitration in pathological conditions characterized by the overproduction of H_2O_2 and NO_2^- or nitric oxide. Further elucidation of the behavior of the heme (iron) on reaction with NO_2^-/H_2O_2 system is essential to the development of therapeutic methods that will focus on the prevention of oxidation and nitration.

The common feature of all putative mechanisms of protein nitration is the direct or indirect dependence of H_2O_2. H_2O_2 is a small, diffusible, and ubiquitous molecule that can be synthesized and destroyed rapidly in response to various stimuli. Apart from its involvement in tyrosine nitration, the H_2O_2 molecule is an intracellular messenger that regulates different signaling pathways [41,42] through stimulation of tyrosine phosphorylation. Thus, the intracellular concentration of H_2O_2 is an important factor in modulation of cardiovascular function. We summarized large number of studies so far and illustrated the "Ying and Yang" dual sides of H_2O_2 in the scheme below. A signaling role for H_2O_2 is now establishing, but many questions remain to be answered. The role of H_2O_2 in different sub-cellular compartments is unclear; The specific H_2O_2 signaling induced by different stimuli still remains to be explored and the interaction between H_2O_2 signalings and its physiologic or pathological consequences are attractive but need more work. The unanswered question is whether the same tyrosines are undergoing nitration while excess endogenous H_2O_2 is produced. If so, the formation of nitrotyrosine interferes with the H_2O_2 –stimulated signaling pathway. What are the possible pathophysiological implications of the heme(Fe)/H_2O_2/NO_2^- nitration system in cardiovascular disease is another question that should be addressed.

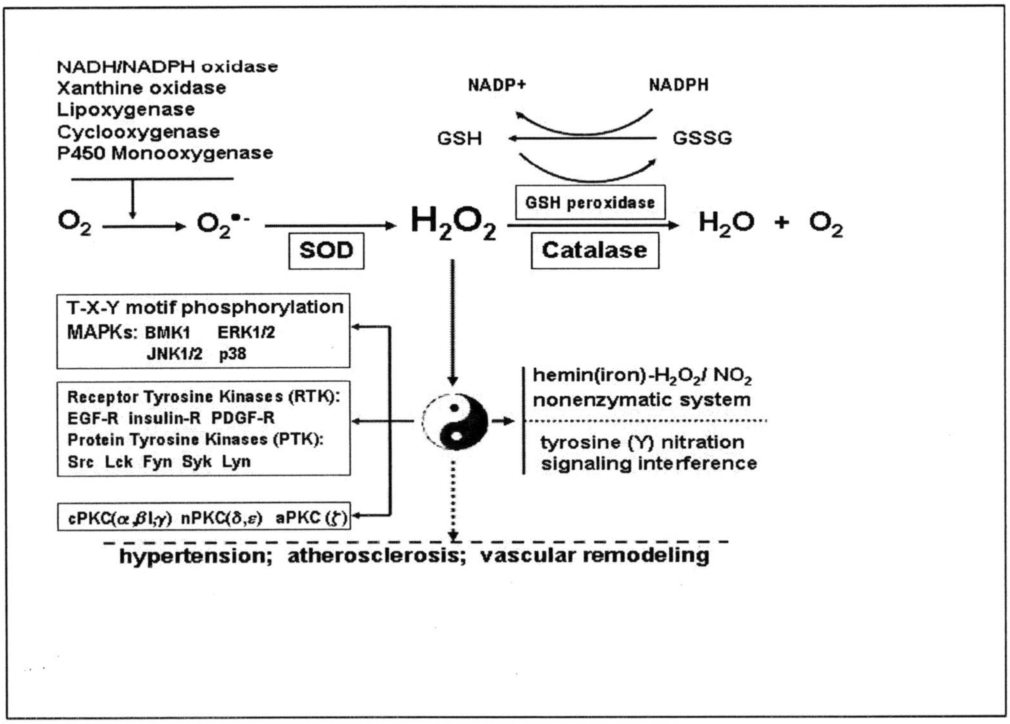

REFERENCES

[1] Willerson JT and Kereiakes DJ. Endothelial dysfunction. *Circulation* 108: 2060-2061, 2003.

[2] Katsuki S, Arnold W, Mittal C and Murad F. Stimulation of guanylate cyclase by sodium nitroprusside, nitroglycerin and nitric oxide in various tissue preparations and comparison to the effects of sodium azide and hydroxylamine. *J Cyclic Nucleotide Res 3*: 23-35, 1977.

[3] Furchgott RF and Zawadzki JV. The obligatory role of endothelial cells in the relaxation of arterial smooth muscle by acetylcholine. *Nature 288*: 373-376, 1980.

[4] Bian K, Davis K, Kuret J, Binder L and Murad F. Nitrotyrosine formation with endotoxin-induced kidney injury detected by immunohistochemistry. *Am J Physiol 277*: F33-40, 1999.

[5] Bian K and Murad F. Diversity of endotoxin-induced nitrotyrosine formation in macrophage-endothelium-rich organs. *Free Radic Biol Med 31*: 421-429, 2001.

[6] Eiserich JP, Hristova M, Cross CE, Jones AD, Freeman BA, Halliwell B and van der Vliet A. Formation of nitric oxide-derived inflammatory oxidants by myeloperoxidase in neutrophils. *Nature 391*: 393-397, 1998.

[7] Turko IV and Murad F. Protein nitration in cardiovascular diseases. *Pharmacol Rev 54*: 619-634, 2002.

[8] Bian K and Murad F. Nitric oxide (NO)--biogeneration, regulation, and relevance to human diseases. *Front Biosci 8*: d264-278, 2003.

[9] Willerson JT. Systemic and local inflammation in patients with unstable atherosclerotic plaques. *Prog Cardiovasc Dis 44*: 469-478, 2002.

[10] Beckmann JS, Ye YZ, Anderson PG, Chen J, Accavitti MA, Tarpey MM and White CR. Extensive nitration of protein tyrosines in human atherosclerosis detected by immunohistochemistry. *Biol Chem Hoppe Seyler 375*: 81-88, 1994.

[11] Evans P, Kaur H, Mitchinson MJ and Halliwell B. Do human atherosclerotic lesions contain nitrotyrosine? *Biochem Biophys Res Commun 226*: 346-351, 1996.

[12] Morton LW, Puddey IB and Croft KD. Comparison of nitration and oxidation of tyrosine in advanced human carotid plaque proteins. *Biochem J 370*: 339-344, 2003.

[13] Sucu N, Unlu A, Tamer L, Aytacoglu B, Ercan B, Dikmengil M and Atik U. 3-Nitrotyrosine in atherosclerotic blood vessels. *Clin Chem Lab Med 41*: 23-25, 2003.

[14] Luoma JS, Stralin P, Marklund SL, Hiltunen TP, Sarkioja T and Yla-Herttuala S. Expression of extracellular SOD and iNOS in macrophages and smooth muscle cells in human and rabbit atherosclerotic lesions: colocalization with epitopes characteristic of oxidized LDL and peroxynitrite-modified proteins. *Arterioscler Thromb Vasc Biol 18*: 157-167, 1998.

[15] Baker CS, Hall RJ, Evans TJ, Pomerance A, Maclouf J, Creminon C, Yacoub MH and Polak JM. Cyclooxygenase-2 is widely expressed in atherosclerotic lesions affecting native and transplanted human coronary arteries and colocalizes with inducible nitric oxide synthase and nitrotyrosine particularly in macrophages. *Arterioscler Thromb Vasc Biol 19*: 646-655, 1999.

[16] Leeuwenburgh C, Hardy MM, Hazen SL, Wagner P, Oh-ishi S, Steinbrecher UP and Heinecke JW. Reactive nitrogen intermediates promote low density lipoprotein oxidation in human atherosclerotic intima. *J Biol Chem 272*: 1433-1436, 1997.

[17] Zou MH, Leist M and Ullrich V. Selective nitration of prostacyclin synthase and defective vasorelaxation in atherosclerotic bovine coronary arteries. *Am J Pathol 154*: 1359-1365, 1999.

[18] Bar-Shavit R, Sabbah V, Lampugnani MG, Marchisio PC, Fenton JW, 2nd, Vlodavsky I and Dejana E. An Arg-Gly-Asp sequence within thrombin promotes endothelial cell adhesion. *J Cell Biol 112*: 335-344, 1991.

[19] Vadseth C, Souza JM, Thomson L, Seagraves A, Nagaswami C, Scheiner T, Torbet J, Vilaire G, Bennett JS, Murciano JC, Muzykantov V, Penn MS, Hazen SL, Weisel JW and Ischiropoulos H. Pro-thrombotic state induced by post translational modification of fibrinogen by reactive nitrogen species. *J Biol Chem*, 2003.

[20] Murad F. Cellular signaling with nitric oxide and cyclic GMP. *Braz J Med Biol Res 32*: 1317-1327, 1999.

[21] Beckman JS. Protein tyrosine nitration and peroxynitrite. *Faseb J 16*: 1144, 2002.

[22] Souza JM, Daikhin E, Yudkoff M, Raman CS and Ischiropoulos H. Factors determining the selectivity of protein tyrosine nitration. *Arch Biochem Biophys 371*: 169-178, 1999.

[23] Wu W, Chen Y and Hazen SL. Eosinophil peroxidase nitrates protein tyrosyl residues. Implications for oxidative damage by nitrating intermediates in eosinophilic inflammatory disorders. *J Biol Chem 274*: 25933-25944, 1999.

[24] Sampson JB, Ye Y, Rosen H and Beckman JS. Myeloperoxidase and horseradish peroxidase catalyze tyrosine nitration in proteins from nitrite and hydrogen peroxide. *Arch Biochem Biophys 356*: 207-213, 1998.

[25] Thukkani AK, McHowat J, Hsu FF, Brennan ML, Hazen SL, Ford DA. Identification of alpha-chloro fatty aldehydes and unsaturated lysophosphatidylcholine molecular species in human atherosclerotic lesions. *Circulation. 108*:3128-3133, 2003.

[26] Augusto O, Bonini MG, Amanso AM, Linares E, Santos CC and De Menezes SL. Nitrogen dioxide and carbonate radical anion: two emerging radicals in biology. *Free Radic Biol Med 32*: 841-859, 2002.

[27] Dunford HB. One-electron oxidations by peroxidases. Xenobiotica 25: 725-733, 1995.

[28] Paoli M, Marles-Wright J and Smith A. Structure-function relationships in heme-proteins. *DNA Cell Biol 21*: 271-280, 2002.

[29] Nelson MJ, Batt DG, Thompson JS and Wright SW. Reduction of the active-site iron by potent inhibitors of lipoxygenases. *J Biol Chem 266*: 8225-8229, 1991.

[30] Poulos TL, Li H and Raman CS. Heme-mediated oxygen activation in biology: cytochrome c oxidase and nitric oxide synthase. *Curr Opin Chem Biol 3*: 131-137, 1999.

[31] Ponka P. Cell biology of heme. *Am J Med Sci 318*: 241-256, 1999.

[32] Asatryan L, Ziouzenkova O, Duncan R and Sevanian A. Heme and lipid peroxides in hemoglobin-modified low-density lipoprotein mediate cell survival and adaptation to oxidative stress. *Blood 102*: 1732-1739, 2003.

[33] Bian K, Gao Z, Weisbrodt N and Murad F. The nature of heme/iron-induced protein tyrosine nitration. *Proc Natl Acad Sci U S A 100*: 5712-5717, 2003.

[34] Isogai Y, Iizuka T and Shiro Y. The mechanism of electron donation to molecular oxygen by phagocytic cytochrome b558. *J Biol Chem 270*: 7853-7857, 1995.

[35] Thomas DD, Espey MG, Vitek MP, Miranda KM and Wink DA. Protein nitration is mediated by heme and free metals through Fenton-type chemistry: an alternative to the NO/O_2- reaction. *Proc Natl Acad Sci U S A 99*: 12691-12696, 2002.

[36] Comporti M. Introduction-serial review: iron and cellular redox status. *Free Radic Biol Med 32*: 565-567, 2002.

[37] Welch KD, Davis TZ and Aust SD. Iron autoxidation and free radical generation: effects of buffers, ligands, and chelators. *Arch Biochem Biophys 397*: 360-369, 2002.

[38] Lovstad RA. A kinetic study of the coupled iron-ceruloplasmin catalyzed oxidation of ascorbate in the presence of albumin. *Biometals 8*: 328-331, 1995.

[39] Fraga CG and Oteiza PI. Iron toxicity and antioxidant nutrients. *Toxicology 180*: 23-32, 2002.

[40] Viner RI, Ferrington DA, Aced GI, Miller-Schlyer M, Bigelow DJ and Schoneich C. In vivo aging of rat skeletal muscle sarcoplasmic reticulum Ca-ATPase. Chemical analysis and quantitative simulation by exposure to low levels of peroxyl radicals. *Biochim Biophys Acta 1329*: 321-335, 1997.

[41] Kamata H and Hirata H. Redox regulation of cellular signalling. *Cell Signal 11*: 1-14, 1999.

[42] Abe MK, Chao TS, Solway J, Rosner MR and Hershenson MB. Hydrogen peroxide stimulates mitogen-activated protein kinase in bovine tracheal myocytes: implications for human airway disease. *Am J Respir Cell Mol Biol 11*: 577-585, 1994.

In: Current Topics in Atherosclerosis Research
Editor: Yong J. Geng, pp. 81-102
ISBN 1-59454-428-X

Chapter V

THROMBOGENESIS AND ANTI-THROMBOGENESIS IN ATHEROSCLEROSIS MEDIATED BY PROSTANOIDS THROUGH THE CYCLOOXYGENASE PATHWAY

Ke-He Ruan**

Vascular Biology Research Center and Division of Hematology, Department of Internal Medicine, The University of Texas Health Science Center, Houston, Texas

ABSTRACT

Atherosclerosis is characterized by the thickening and obstruction of the arterial lumen and thrombosis. There is growing evidence that the components of the hemostatic system, thrombogenesis and vascular inflammation play significant roles in the development and progression of atherosclerosis and its complications. Prostanoids (which belong to the eicosanoids), thromboxane A_2 (TXA_2), prostacyclin (PGI_2), and prostaglandin E_2 (PGE_2) synthesized through the cyclooxygenase (COX) pathway are the most potent molecules that mediate thrombogenesis, anti-thrombogenesis, and vascular inflammation, respectively. Understanding the biosynthesis and action mechanisms of TXA_2, PGI_2, and PGE_2 are key steps toward preventing atherosclerosis and developing new therapeutic strategies. This chapter summarizes the current advances in biosynthesis and signaling of the prostanoids that mediate the pathophyological processes of thrombogenesis, anti-thrombogenesis, and the vascular inflammation in developing and

* Correspondence concerning this article should be addressed to Ke-He Ruan, M.D., Ph.D., Division of Hematology, Department of Internal Medicine, University of Texas Health Science Center at Houston, 6431 Fannin St., Houston, Texas 77030. (Tel.: 713-500-6769, Fax: 713-500-6810, Email: kruan@uth.tmc.edu).

preventing atherosclerosis and their effects in acute thrombosis and myocardial infarctions.

Color graphics are presented at the end of the chapter.

Keywords: Atherosclerosis, Cyclooxygenase, Prostaglandin, Prostanoid, and Thromboxane

CYCLOOXYGENASE AND ATHEROSCLEROSIS

Atherosclerotic disease is recognized as a chronic inflammatory disorder with variable phases of cellular proliferation and thrombotic activity in arteries. The linkage of inflammation and thrombogenesis associated with atherogenesis is widely recognized and described in numerous chapters. As a simple description, the vascular endothelium is a large organ that secretes various factors regulating vascular inflammation and tone, cellular growth, platelet and leukocyte interactions, and thrombogenesis. Endothelial dysfunction is an early event in atherogenesis and is also important in establishing coronary artery disease [1]. Platelets and their interaction with vessel walls, which contribute to atherosclerosis through thrombosis, platelet aggregation, vasoconstriction, local vascular inflammatory response, and in the formation of the coronary thrombus, are caused by endothelial dysfunctions regulated by many lipid metabolites, including prostanoids. The biosynthesis of prostanoids, including TXA_2, PGI_2 and PGE_2, is regulated by the functional coupling of COX isoform-1 (COX-1) or isoform-2 (COX-2) with its downstream synthases. Functional coupling of COX-1 with TXA_2 synthase (TXAS) mediates TXA_2 synthesis in platelets, which is a potent vasoconstrictor and platelet aggregative agonist. In contrast, both COX-1 and COX-2 coupled to PGI_2 synthase (PGIS) mediates the production of endothelial PGI_2, a vasodilator that inhibits platelet aggregation against thrombogenesis. In addition, COX-2 is inducible and functionally couples to PGE_2 synthase (PGES) to produce PGE_2, a pro-inflammatory factor contributing to vascular inflammation during the development of atherosclerosis. Since COX-2 is up-regulated in activated monocytes/macrophages that play key roles in the pathogenesis of atherosclerosis, a relationship between COX-2 and atherosclerosis has been proposed [2]. Unfortunately, it is not a simple cause-and-effect model due to conflicting data in the use of COX-2 inhibitors in clinical and experimental observations.

COX-2 can be induced by proinflammatory mediators, including interleukin-1 (IL-1), tumor necrosis factor (TNF), interferon-α, free radicals, endotoxin, platelet-derived growth factor, hypoxia, and sheer stress [3], and also expressed in vascular inflammation sites implicated in the development of atherosclerosis [3-5]. COX-2 is present in cells that comprise the atheromatous lesion, and the COX-2-mediated end-products of prostaglandins, such as PGE_2 are increased in atherosclerosis similar to that seen in other inflammatory conditions [3,6]. It is particularly relevant that COX-2 expression is found in human atheromatous plaque lesions in diseased coronary arteries removed at the time of surgical revascularization, but *not* in normal coronary arteries [4-5]. This evidence emphasizes the vascular inflammation nature of atherosclerosis, which has lead to treatment with COX-2 inhibitors as an action to reduce the pathological process of atherosclerosis. Indeed, some experiments have confirmed this hypothesis in which the COX-2 inhibitor could reduce the early atherosclerosis in LDL-receptor deficient mice [7]. This study supports the use of COX-2 inhibitors as an anti-inflammatory approach for the prevention and treatment of atherosclerosis. However, COX-2 inhibitors can reduce PGI_2 production in the endothelium and leave only TXA_2 production in platelets, promoting the pathological processes of platelet aggregation and thrombosis. This imbalance between TXA_2 and PGI_2 may not only promote the implications of atherosclerosis, but also trigger coronary artery diseases [8]. The VIGOR trial demonstrated a five-fold increase in the incidence of myocardial infarction in the rofecoxib (COX-2 inhibitor)-treated group compared to the naproxen (a traditional NSAID drug)-treated group [8-9]. Thus, selective COX-2 inhibition may not offer cardiovascular protection as aspirin-like drugs do [8-10]. Therefore, it is obvious that many remaining questions must be answered before the role of COX-2 in the atherosclerotic process is understood. The discussion of the current advances in the functional coupling of COX-1 and -2 and their downstream synthases that mediate the biosynthesis of TXA_2, PGI_2 and PGE_2, which play key roles in thrombogenesis, anti-thrombogenesis and vascular inflammation associated with atherosclerosis development, will provide a more comprehensive understanding of the roles of COX-mediated pathophysiological processes in atherosclerosis.

TXA_2 IN ATHEROSCLEROSIS

Thrombogenesis in Atherosclerosis

Recently, the hypothesis of intracoronary thrombosis being triggered by plaque ulceration or fissuration, has gained wide acceptance as one of the key events in the pathophysiology of acute coronary syndromes. In the last few years, the intracoronary thrombosis in the atherosclerotic coronary arteries, triggered by plaque ulceration, is involved in key mechanisms during myocardial ischemia, and has been recognized as one of the key events in the pathophysiological process of acute coronary syndromes in patients. One of the mechanisms ensues following arterial injury and/or plaque ulceration, platelets are activated and adhere to the damaged vessel wall, therefore releasing large amounts of TXA_2 mediated vasoconstriction and platelet-aggregation. Platelet-induced coronary vasoconstriction may therefore contribute to the occurrence of heart attacks [11].

The action of TXA_2-mediated thrombogenesis in developing atherosclerosis and coronary artery diseases is not only regulated by the biosynthesis of TXA_2 through the COX pathway, but is also regulated by TXA_2 signaling through its specific receptor. Elucidation of the biosynthesis and action mechanisms of TXA_2 and their controlling factors at cellular and molecular levels are important to reveal the fundamental issues of developing atherosclerosis and coronary artery diseases. In the past decade, COX pathway studies have greatly advanced our knowledge of TXA_2 biosynthesis, metabolism, signaling and modulation, which have provided clues for the development of therapeutic strategies for the prevention and treatment of atherosclerosis and coronary artery diseases.

Biosynthesis of TXA_2 and other Prostanoids through the COX Pathway

Fig. 1 outlines the biosynthesis of prostanoids including thromboxane and prostaglandins formed via the COX pathway from arachidonic acid (AA) in three steps [12-16]: (a) stimulus-induced mobilization of AA from membrane phosphoglycerides by cytosolic phospholipase A_2 ($cPLA_2$); (b) conversion of AA to the prostaglandin endoperoxide, prostaglandin H_2 (PGH_2), by COX-1 or -2 (COX-2); and (c) isomerization of PGH_2 to biologically active end-products, prostanoids (including prostaglandin D_2 (PGD_2), E_2 (PGE_2), F_2 (PGF_2), and I_2 (prostacyclin, PGI_2) or TXA_2), by individual synthases in tissue specific manners. Prostanoids act as local hormones in the vicinity of their production sites to regulate hemostasis, smooth muscle functions and other diverse biological functions, which are mainly mediated by specific prostanoid receptors in the plasma membrane (Fig. 2).

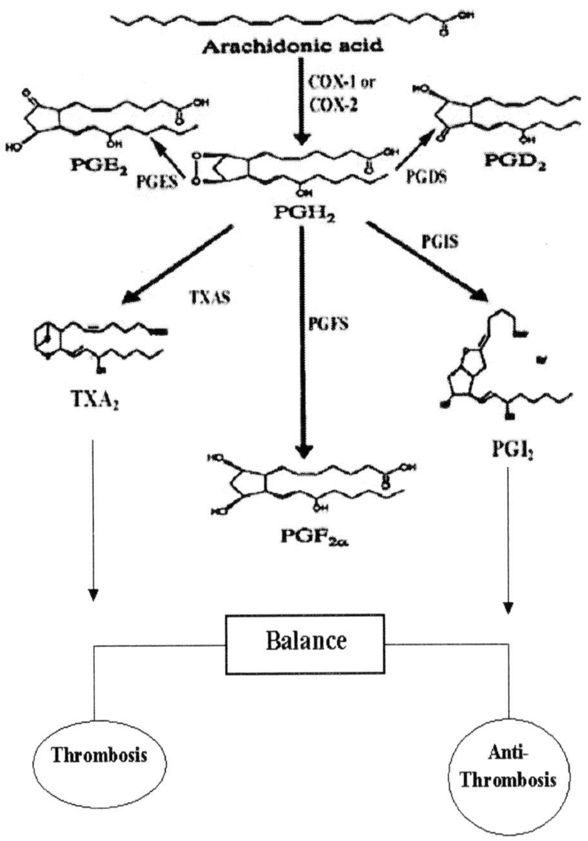

Figure 1. Biosynthetic pathways for prostanoid formation. The unbalancing functions between TXA2 and PGI2 is one of the key factors involved in atherosclerosis and its complications.

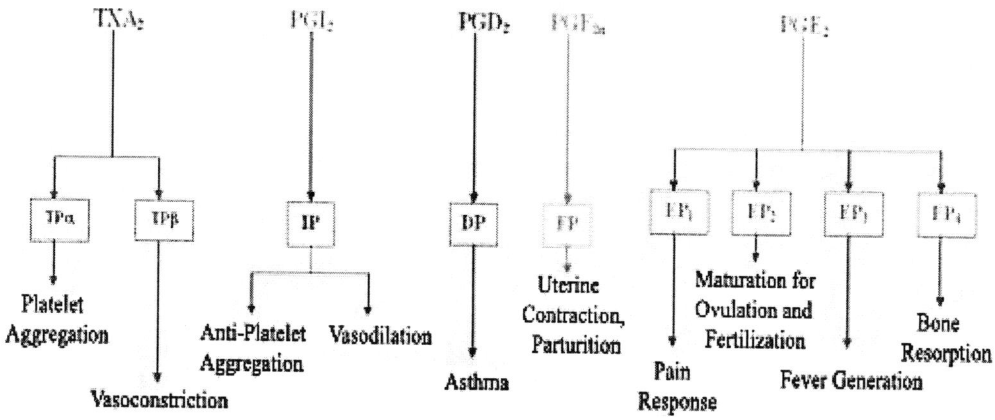

Figure 2. Biological functions of the prostanoids mediated by their specific receptors. The receptors of PGD_2, PGE_2, $PGF_{2\alpha}$, PGI_2 or TXA_2 are termed DP, EP, FP, IP and TP, respectively. Four subtype EPs are termed EP1, EP2, EP3 and EP4.

Functional Coupling of COX-1 and TXAS in the Biosynthesis of TXA_2

COX-1 [17] and COX-2 [18] have been cloned, crystallized and well characterized in their structures and functions. The TXAS gene has been cloned from different sources [19-21], and its synthase is characterized as a microsomal cytochrome P450 by optical and electron paramagnetic resonance (EPR) spectroscopy. However, the synthase lacks the monooxygenase activity found in other P450s [22-23]. Like many other mammalian microsomal P450s, TXAS is located on the endoplasmic reticulum (ER) membrane. The accumulation of discoveries in the biosynthesis of prostanoids has advanced our knowledge at the cellular and molecular levels. It is known that COX-1 is a housekeeping enzyme coupled to TXAS and PGIS to generate balanced amounts of TXA_2 and PGI_2 (Figure 1) and to regulate the normal hemostatic and vascular functions in pathophysiological conditions. On the other hand, the inducible COX-2 is favored to couple with PGIS rather than TXAS.

The biosynthesis of TXA_2 from AA resulting from arterial injury and/or plaque ulceration in the atherosclerotic artery occurs instantly through the efficient coordination of COX-1 with TXAS in the ER membrane. The detailed crystallographic structure of the detergent-solubilized COX-1 has been used to build a membrane topology model in which the catalytic domains of the proteins lie on the lumenal side of the ER and are anchored to the ER membrane by hydrophobic side chains of the amphipathic helices A-D [17-18]. These hydrophobic side chains of the membrane anchor domains also form an entrance to the substrate-binding channel and can potentially form an initial docking site for the lipid substrate, AA [17-18].

Despite the fact that COX enzymes have been well characterized at the 3D structural level, little information is available about the cellular and molecular factors controlling the functional coupling between COX-1 and TXAS in the native membrane-bound environment. No crystal structure is available for any eicosanoid-synthesizing P450s thus far. It is also unknown how the reaction occurs in coordination within the ER membrane. However, the belief that all P450s possess similar backbone structures with multiple helices and a conserved Cys residue bound to the heme iron lead to the obtainment of a working 3D model of TXAS by the homology modeling approach using the crystal structures of $P450_{BM-3}$ [24] as a template after TXAS cDNA was cloned [25]. The model structure has provided many clues for the membrane topology and structure/function relationship in coordination with COX in the biosynthesis of TXA_2.

An active site of human TXAS has been proposed by model-guided mutagenesis [26]. The most important information is that the membrane topology model from recent studies elucidated the relationship between the ER membrane and the TXAS protein. It is believed that the large cytoplasmic polypeptide of TXAS is anchored to the ER membrane by its N-terminal hydrophobic domain and a few residues in the F/G loop. The active site of TXAS is in the cytoplasmic side of the ER membrane. This allows my laboratory to hypothesize a coordination model between COX-1 and TXAS in the ER membrane (Figure 3). In the coupling reaction of COX and TXAS, PGH_2 produced by the COX-1 in the ER lumen, must pass through the ER membrane barrier to the catalytic site of TXAS on the cytoplasmic side of the ER membrane (Figure 3). The factors that influence the delivery of PGH_2 from COX-1 to TXAS in the ER membrane are not clearly addressed. However, it is a target of new drug designs for specifically blocking COX-1/TXAS coupling in the biosynthesis of TXA_2 mediated thrombogenesis in atherosclerosis.

Receptors of TXA_2 and other Prostanoids

TXA_2 acts as a local hormone in its production site to regulate hemostasis and smooth muscle functions in response to initial atherosclerosis and coronary artery damages, which is mediated by specific receptors in the plasma membrane of the cells similar to other prostanoids [27-28, Figure 2). To understand how TXA_2 mediates thrombosis and vasoconstriction in atherosclerosis and coronary artery diseases, a basic understanding of TXA_2 receptor properties and its relationship with other prostanoid receptor properties is vitally important.

The prostanoid receptors are classified into five basic types based on their cognate prostanoid (PGD_2, PGE_2, $PGF_{2\alpha}$, PGI_2 or TXA_2) and are termed DP, EP, FP, IP, and TP receptors, respectively (Figure 2). In addition, the EP receptors are subdivided into four subtypes (EP1, EP2, EP3 and EP4) based on the different signaling responses to PGE_2 (Figure 2). Human TPα receptor was first purified from a platelet in 1989 and the cDNA was cloned from placenta in 1991 [28]. Other human prostanoid receptor cDNAs, including those for IP, DP, FP, EP1, EP2, EP3, and EP4 have also been cloned, and their primary biologic functions have been identified [29-37]. Prostanoid receptors can be divided into two functional groups using smooth muscle assays: relaxant receptors (including DP, EP2, EP4, and IP) and excitatory receptors (including EP1, FP, and TP).

Another form of TP receptor, termed as TPβ was also cloned in 1994, which is encoded by the same gene as the TPα receptor [33]. TP receptors in platelet and placenta are commonly referred to as the TPα (first cloned) receptor, and the receptors in endothelium and vascular smooth muscle are referred to as the TPβ receptor [33]. The TP isoforms are identical in the first 328 residues, but differ in their C-terminal domains. TPα and TPβ receptors have 15 and 79 residues within their unique C-tail sequences, respectively [33]. TPβ couples to the same Gq of the G protein family as the TPα; however, their unique C-tail sequences may be involved in determining Gs or Gi coupling and may act as a determinant of receptor-G-protein coupling efficiency.

The biological function of the TP receptor to mediate hemostasis and vascular function has been further confirmed by recent gene-knockout experiments. The TP-knockout mice show normal organ development. However, thromboxane agonist binding cannot be detected in tissues. In the hemostasis test, bleeding times of TP-deficient mice were prolonged and their platelets do not aggregate after exposure to TXA_2 agonists. Aggregation responses after collagen stimulation are also delayed. In the hemodynamic test, infusion of the TP agonist, U-46619, causes an increase in blood pressure followed by cardiovascular collapse in wild-type mice, but U-46619 caused no hemodynamic effect in TP-deficient mice. AA can significantly reduce blood pressure in TP-deficient mice. It can be concluded that TP-deficient mice have a bleeding disorder and an altered vascular responses to TXA_2 and AA. Most of the recognized functions of TXA_2 are mediated by the single known *Tp* gene [38-41].

Action Mechanism of the TP Receptor

As with the cloning of most prostanoid receptors, the emphasis of early studies on pharmacological functions has extended to the molecular mechanisms of specific prostanoid recognition, G protein coupling, and signal transduction. Structure/function relationship studies of prostanoid receptors have become one of the most challenging fields in eicosanoid research.

For over a decade, structural and functional studies of prostanoid receptors have focused on the identification of the specific sites for ligand binding and G protein coupling.

All known prostanoid receptors belong to the rhodopsin-type G protein-coupled receptor (GPCR) super-family, which has seven conserved TM domains. The diverse and/or opposite biological functions of the individual prostanoid receptors are mediated by selective ligand binding on the extracellular side of the membrane and interaction with different heterotrimeric G proteins on the intracellular side [28]. Based on the G protein coupling mechanism, prostanoid receptors can be grouped into three categories: (1) the DP, EP2, EP4, and IP receptors are coupled to the stimulation of adenylate cyclase to increase cAMP as the second messenger; (2) the EP1, FP, and TP receptors are coupled to calcium mobilization by increasing intracellular calcium levels as second messengers; (3) and the EP3 receptor is coupled to the inhibition of adenylate cyclase to decrease cAMP production [42].

The homology alignment-based mutagenesis studies of the transmembrane (TM) domains of the TP and other prostanoid receptors have suggested that the conserved regions in the third and seventh TM domains are involved in binding the core structure of TXA_2, which consists of a carboxylic acid, a hydroxyl group on carbon 15, and two aliphatic side chains [42-44]. However, residues in the TM domains are highly conserved in all known prostanoid receptors, and therefore probably do not define the differences among the receptors in specific interactions with ligands. Thus, the involvement of the extracellular loop (eLP) domains of prostanoid receptors in the selective ligand recognition, similar to some other GPCRs, has been focused upon [45-48]. However, interpretation of the data on the eLP specific determinants among prostanoid receptors is limited by the lack of experimental 3D structural information for the extramembrane domains.

Due to the difficulty of membrane protein crystallization, rhodopsin is the only GPCR whose crystal structure has been determined thus far [49-52]. The crystal structure of rhodopsin offers a structural template for the conserved TM helices of other GPCRs, including the prostanoid receptors. Nevertheless, the rhodopsin crystal structure provides few structural clues for the extracellular and intracellular domains of the prostanoid receptors, due to the very different segment lengths and primary sequences. The lack of the 3D structural models on the prostanoid receptors has become a major obstacle for further investigation of their molecular mechanisms and in the designs of pharmacological intervention strategies.

Recently, my laboratory has integrated high-resolution NMR techniques with general biochemical and molecular biological approaches to advance the structure/function relationship studies of the human TP receptor. These studies have made significant advances in this field. Through the development of an approach combining 2D NMR spectroscopy and recombinant protein techniques, the TP eLP_2 residues involved in the antagonist (SQ29,548) recognition were first identified [48,53-54]. This structural information was supported by results from other groups using traditional biochemical and molecular approaches, such as affinity labeling [47] and site-directed mutagenesis [45-46]. Our NMR 3D structural model of the TP antagonist/receptor interaction was able to interpret some important earlier observations which had been puzzling. The structural features of the dynamic conformation of the eLP_2, controlled by the disulfide bond, provides a mechanism for the oxidation/reduction regulation of the TP receptor ligand binding activity reported in 1990 [55], and for the results from the mutation studies of Cys residues in TP eLP_1 and eLP_2 done by Dorn's and Tai's groups [45,55-56]. The involvement of multiple loops in forming the ligand pocket, shown by the NMR 3D structure of the eLPs, explains earlier observations that ligand binding activities of prostanoid receptors are affected by the mutation of residues in different eLPs, even residues far away from the direct ligand contact sites. This is because the distal residues affect the loop arrangement and conformation, which leads to changes in the shape and size of the ligand recognition pocket for ligand docking.

Despite the fact that the TP antagonist (SQ29,548) recognition pocket has been partially defined, there is still the question of how the receptor distinguishes antagonist from agonist. As evidenced by several research groups, the binding sites for agonist and antagonists on the TP receptor are different. Mayeux et al provided evidence that changes in the pH affected the binding affinities of agonist and antagonist differently [57]. The TP receptor W299L mutant lost binding activity to an antagonist but still bound the agonist [43]. Studies by Dorn et al using chimeric proteins also indicated that the binding sites of the agonist and antagonist are distinct [58]. These studies prompted for further definition of the agonist recognition site in the TP eLPs. The differences in the ligand recognition sites for the TP agonist and antagonist can be identified by the comparison of the residues involved in the two types of ligand recognition.

It is no longer a question of whether the structure/function studies of TP receptor will provide molecular information that is beneficial to design specific TP receptor inhibitors for the preventive and therapeutic uses in atherosclerosis and coronary artery diseases. Many TP receptor modulators have been developed and are being tested [59].

PGI_2 IN ATHEROSCLEROSIS

PGI_2 and Atherosclerosis

As mentioned earlier, PGI_2 produced by the COX pathway is a major prostaglandin produced by endothelial cells as a potent inhibitor of leukocyte activation and adhesion, platelet aggregation, and vascular smooth muscle cell proliferation, migration, and contraction [7,14]. It is also well evidenced by different researches that PGI_2 production is increased in activated monocyte/macrophages, which play a key role in inflammation as the pathogenesis of atherosclerosis. In clinical trials, increasing levels of PGI_2 are associated with patients with 'activated platelet' conditions such as unstable atherosclerotic disease as well as post vascular interventional procedures [11,60]. On one hand, it would not be unreasonable to predict a facilitative role for COX-2 in these conditions of increased PGI_2 production, given its inducible nature and the fact that COX-2 is responsible for the majority of PGI_2 produced in the body [61]. On the other hand, nonselective NSAID therapy (sulindac and indomethacin) inhibits initial proliferation and prevents or slows vascular changes in atherosclerosis-prone mice while aspirin and nimesulide (a selective COX-2 inhibitor) do not [62-63]. Compared with nitric oxide, PGI_2 is more directed against TXA_2 to protect the platelet-endothelial interaction. It is one of the major factors to prevent the development of atherosclerosis and platelet calation-based coronary artery diseases. It is not a question about understanding the biosynthesis of PGI_2 through the COX pathway, but rather the functional coupling of COX-2 and PGIS in atherosclerosis and PGI_2 signaling through its receptor that are extremely valuable for the developing strategies for protection from atherosclerosis and its implications.

Biosynthesis of PGI_2 Through the COX Pathway

The general pathway of PGI_2 biosynthesis is similar with TXA_2 described in Figure 1. However, TXA_2 synthesis occurs in platelets and PGI_2 synthesis mainly occurs in endothelial and smooth muscle cells. The endothelium participates in the regulation of blood flow and tonus of the vascular wall, activation of thrombocytes, adhesion of monocytes to the vascular wall, thrombogenesis, lipid metabolism, and growth of vessels, which are important to regulate atherosclerosis. Endothelial cells may produce some 25 different biologically active substances. PGI_2 is one of the most abundant substances. Under physiological conditions, endothelial cells release a small amount of PGI_2 through the functional coupling of PGIS and COX-1 in the cells. The amount of PGI_2 can be detected in the circulation from large arteries to small capillaries [64]. Recently, PGI_2 production in female reproductive tissues has been documented. PGI_2 is present at the embryo implantation site and in human fallopian tubes [65-66].

Functional Coupling of COX-2 and PGIS in the Biosynthesis of PGI_2

A number of pathophysiological stimuli, e.g. a rise of the blood pressure, drop of the partial oxygen pressure, the action of acetylcholine, ADP, ATP, thrombin, bradykinin or histamine, inflammatory mediators, growth factors and hormones and artery injuries can increase PGI_2 production. It has been demonstrated that the increasing PGI_2 production is associated with the increasing expression of the inducible COX-2 in the cells. It has been observed that COX-2 contributed substantially to PGI_2-synthesis in patients with atherosclerosis. Thus, the induced PGI_2 synthesis in atherosclerosis through functional coupling of COX-2 and PGIS has been proposed and widely accepted.

It is more interesting that in human vascular smooth muscle cells, the prostacyclin-mimetic iloprost could up-regulate COX-2 mRNA and protein. It is concluded, that the observed up-regulation of COX-2 with subsequent release of newly synthesized PGI_2 provides a positive feedback of prostaglandins on their own synthesizing enzyme. This might be important for control of atherosclerosis through the controls of proliferation, migration and differentiation as well as inhibition of platelet aggregation by the newly synthesized PGI_2 [67]. The characterization of the COX-2/PGIS coupling in atherosclerosis is important to the preventive and therapeutic strategies today because the roles of benefits and risks involved in taking COX-2 inhibitors for atherosclerosis needs to be addressed. It also represents one of the major challenges in atherosclerosis research.

Little information is available for the understanding of the cellular and molecular mechanisms of the functional coupling between COX-2 and PGIS in the cells at the atherosclerosis site. Many attempts have been made to address the critical issues. Our current cellular and molecular studies for the coupling have revealed some important mechanism about the functional coupling occurring in the cells. As described above, PGIS belongs to the eicosanoid-synthesizing cytochrome P450s, similar to TXAS located in the ER membrane. The biosynthesis of PGI_2 requires the efficient coordination of PGIS with COX-1 or -2 localized in the ER lumen. Understanding the membrane topology of the catalytic portion of PGIS with respect to the ER membrane can help to elucidate the coupling mechanism in the membrane for the biosynthesis of PGI_2. Very recently, the membrane topology of the catalytic portion of PGIS, using molecular modeling-guided site-specific antibodies, has been characterized. A working 3-D model of PGIS was constructed by homology modeling using the $P450_{BM-3}$ and 2C5 crystal structures as templates [68-70]. Different site-specific antibodies were used to determine the overall arrangement of the PGIS polypeptide with respect to the ER membrane by immunocytochemistry techniques in cells [69]. These results have provided direct experimental evidences supporting a topological model of PGIS in the ER membrane, in which PGIS is largely exposed on the cytoplasmic side of the ER membrane and anchored to the membrane by its hydrophobic N-terminal domain and some residues in the F/G loop. It has led to the conclusion that the PGIS substrate, PGH_2, produced by the COXs in the ER lumen must pass through the ER membrane barrier to the catalytic site of PGIS on the cytoplasmic side of the ER membrane and be allowed to further characterize PGH_2 moving (presentation) from COXs to PGIS in the cells.

To understand the coordination of COXs with PGIS in the ER membrane, how the presentation of PGH_2 from the COXs to the PGIS substrate access channel occurs in the ER membrane needs to be characterized. The accessibility of the PGIS substrate channel opening to site-specific antibodies for the characterization of its relationship with respect to the membrane has been explored. The working model was used to predict surface portions near the substrate access channel opening. Two peptides corresponding to the surface immediately near the substrate access channel opening and two other peptides corresponding to the surfaces, approximately 10-20 Å (1 Å=0.1 nm) away from the opening, were used to prepare site-specific antibodies. The site-specific antibodies were used to probe the accessibility of the substrate access channel opening in the cells expressing human PGIS. The observations support that the PGIS substrate access channel opening is positioned close to and opens to the ER membrane for quick acceptance of membrane-soluble PGH_2, from the ER membrane or COXs [70].

These results provided experimental evidence for the proposal of a coordination model for the COXs and PGIS in the ER membrane, in which hydrophobic PGH_2 produced from AA by the COXs, is released to the ER membrane and presented to the substrate access channel of PGIS through the ER lipid membrane without leaving the membrane and avoiding the degradation in an aqueous environment. This is a highly efficient way to use the unstable PGH_2 in the native membrane-bound environment. It can be used to explain the mechanisms of the quick response of PGI_2 production when cells are stimulated by the pathophysiological factors under the coordination of COX-2 and PGIS in the membrane. It also implies that beside the tissue specific distribution of PGIS and other downstream synthases, the factors (such as co-localization, and physical approximations of the catalytic sites between COX-2 and its downstream synthases) facilitated by PGH_2 presentation from COX-2 to PGIS may play an important role in controlling specifically functional coupling of COX-2 with PGIS rather than with TXAS.

Signaling of PGI_2

The function of PGI_2 is mainly mediated by the PGI_2 receptor (IP) on the cell surface. The human IP receptor has been cloned [71-72]. The receptor consists of 386 amino acid residues with a predicted molecular mass of roughly 41kD and belongs to the G-protein coupling receptor super family similar to the TP receptor as described in section 2-4. In signaling studies, in addition to the coupling of the IP receptor to Gs α-subunit of the G protein leading to an increase of cAMP production, some reports have also indicated that the IP receptor may also couple to other subtype G proteins. Northern blot analysis and in situ hybridization experiments on human tissues have revealed that IP receptor mRNA is abundantly expressed in the aorta, lung, atrium, ventricle and kidney. These studies have lead to a better understanding of the significance of PGI_2 in humans and will further facilitate the clinical application of PGI_2 [72].

The long proposed role of PGI_2 as an endogenous anti-thrombotic agent has been confirmed by the experimental evidences of IP receptor-knockout in mice. IP-deficient mice develop normally without vascular problems in normal situations. However, an enhanced thrombotic tendency was observed when endothelial damage occurred. These findings also indicated that the anti-thrombotic system mediated by PGI_2 is activated in response to vascular injury to minimize its effects. Further useful information was also obtained from the gene-knockout experiment, in which the IP-deficient mice showed a decreased response to acetic acid-induced writhing test (pain model), indicating that the IP receptor is also involved in mediating pain responses. This suggests that IP receptor is involved in mediating inflammatory pain through sensitizing the free end of sensory neurons and also acting in the spinal cord and brain [38-40].

It has been reported that IP receptor-defect in platelets with pathogenetic significance for development of atherosclerosis in early age. The evidence came from a discovery of a 10 year-old girl diagnosed as an occlusion of the left popliteal artery with a defect of the IP receptor. This defect seems to be genetically determined and might have contributed to the development of atherosclerosis [73].

Recently, in the course of searching for the IP receptor in the brain, a novel subtype, designated as IP-2 was reported by use of the specific ligand (15R)-16-m-tolyl-17,18,19,20-tetranorisocarbacyclin (15R-TIC) and specifically localized in the rostral part of the brain [74]. However, the molecular identity has not been confirmed.

PGI_2 as a Ligand for Nuclear Hormone Receptor-PPAR

In 1990, Issemann & Green reported the discovery of Peroxisome proliferatory-activated receptor (PPAR) [75]. So far, the three isoforms PPARα, β/δ and γ have been cloned and implicated in the regulation of the expression of genes involved in lipid metabolism. In skeletal and cardiac muscle cells it has been demonstrated that the metabolic conversion of fatty acids is controlled by PPARs. In eicosanoids, PGI_2 as an important ligand for PPARδ has been found recently. PGI_2 and its agonists, carbaprostacyclin and iloprost, can effectively induce DNA binding and transcriptional activation by PPARδ. PGI_2, as a ligand for PPARδ mediated vascular functions, was evidenced by the observation of the PPARδ expression increase in rat arteries after balloon injury, which suggests that functions of PGI_2 on vasodilation and anti-platelet aggregation might mediated by the IP receptor and PPARδ [76]. It is more interesting that PGI_2 as a ligand for PPARδ effects on vascular inflammation in atherosclerosis has been proposed recently. The model indicates that the binding of the ligand to the PPARδ may lead to the release of BCL-6, a transcriptional repressor of inflammation. This may result in decreased expression of inflammatory cytokine genes, reduced inflammation, and a decrease in atherosclerosis. Alternatively, in the absence of the ligand, BCL-6 may remain bound to PPARδ, resulting in a pro-inflammatory response [77]. These directly address the relationship of PGI_2 and anti-thrombogenesis and atherosclerosis.

PGE_2 IN ATHEROSCLEROSIS

Vascular Inflammation Mediated by PGE_2 and Atherosclerosis

It is believed that chronic inflammatory processes contribute to the development of atherosclerosis [78]. In this section, the molecular basis of PGE_2 mediated vascular inflammation is discussed. Atherosclerosis involves chronic vascular inflammation mediated by pro-inflammatory molecules such as cytokines, chemokines, adhesion molecules, growth factors, and others [79]. These factors can also induce COX-2 expression and PGE_2 production in the atherosclerosis site. It is particularly interesting that recent studies have implicated a role for PGE_2-dependent matrix metalloproteinase (MMP) biosynthesis in the rupture of an atherosclerotic plaque. Production of MMP-2 and MMP-9 by macrophages has been shown to occur through a PGE_2/cAMP–dependent pathway [79]. Signaling through this pathway involves the functional coupling of COX-2 and PGES in the biosynthesis of PGE_2 and its receptor. Thus, understanding the biosynthesis, functional coupling of COX-2 and PGES and the action mechanisms of the EP receptor isoforms will provide fundamental information for understanding the pathophysiological processes of the vascular inflammation in atherosclerosis mediated by PGE_2.

Biosynthesis of PGE_2

The biosynthesis of PGE_2 through the COX pathway has been summarized in Figure 1. For PGE_2 synthase (PGES), despite the many attempts that have been made to isolate the synthase over the past decades, few molecular aspects have been discovered until recently. The recombinant human microsomal PGES-1 (mPGES-1), which has an identified sequence, was reported in 1999 [80] as a member of the MAPEG (membrane-associated protein in eicosanoid and glutathione metabolism) superfamily with a molecular weight of about 17 kD (152 residues). It represents other groups of eicosanoid-synthesizing enzymes different from the P450 enzymes of TXAS and PGIS with molecular weights about 60 kD. Recently, several other groups have also confirmed the identity of mPGES-1 and found that mPGES-1 is an inducible form of PGES [80], and shares high similarities with MGST-1 (microsomal glutathione S-transfersa-1) in the primary and secondary structures [80]. At the same time, a non-inducible cytosolic PGES (cPGES) was also purified and characterized [81]. Very recently, a third PGES, which shows a broad specificity of thiol requirements, was purified from the microsomal fraction of a bovine heart [82], and the entire sequence of both human and monkey enzymes was determined [82]. This enzyme, designated mPGES-2, has an N-terminal hydrophobic domain followed by a glutaredoxin or thioredoxin homology region [82].

Functional Coupling of COX-2 and mPGES-1 in Atherosclerosis

The induction of COX-2 in monocytes and the resulting production of PGE_2 have been shown to be involved in MMP production by these cells [79]. Simultaneous induction of COX-2 and PGE synthase (PGES) by inflammatory stimuli might modulate the production of MMP by macrophages into atherosclerotic plaques. An enhanced MMP production by macrophages in symptomatic carotid plaques has been evidenced by the enhancement in PGE_2 synthesis as a result of the induction of the functionally coupled inducible COX/PGES [83]. Over-expression of functionally coupled COX-2 and PGES in symptomatic atherosclerotic plaques as one of the basic factors in plaque instability has also been evidenced by the characterization of the expression of COX-2 and PGES in carotid plaques and to correlate it with the extent of inflammatory infiltration and MMP activity and with clinical features of patients' presentation. A study demonstrated the co-localization of COX-2 and PGES in symptomatic lesions has also provided evidence that the synthesis of COX-2 and PGES by activated macrophages associated with acute ischemic syndromes through metalloproteinase-induced plaque rupture. Thus, the identification of pathways that regulate vascular inflammation mediated by the functional coupling of COX-2 and PGES is critical to the formulation of strategies that may reduce vascular inflammation and stabilize plaques in the future.

To date, it is believed that two PGE_2 biosynthesis routes exists, which includes the pathway of the constitutive COX-1/cPGES coupling and the inducible COX-2/mPGES-1 coupling in the cells, even though COX-1/mPGES-1 coupling can occur if a large amount of AA is supplied [82]. The biosynthesis and functions of PGE_2 produced from the different COX/PGES coupling have been characterized to indicate that PGE_2 produced via the two separated biosynthetic pathways may be linked to various physiological and pathological events. For example, in the immediate response elicited by Ca^{2+} agonists, AA is rapidly released by $cPLA_2$ [82] and metabolized to PGE_2 via the constitutive enzymes COX-1 and cPGES. In the delayed response induced by proinflammatory stimuli, AA was slowly and continuously released by $cPLA_2$ and metabolized to PGE_2 via the two inducible enzymes of COX-2 and mPGES-1.

A recent mPGES-1 gene targeting study clearly demonstrated that COX-2-mediated PGE_2 production by lipopolysaccharide-stimulated mouse macrophages depends largely on this enzyme [80]. The expression of mPGES-1 *in vivo* has been reported to be associated with various physiological and pathological events beside inflammation, such as cancer and reproduction [80]. The vascular inflammation in atherosclerosis mediated by COX-2 is likely the result of functional coupling with mPGES-1.

It is primarily interesting that mPGES-1 and PGIS share COX-2 in their functional coupling in the biosynthesis of PGE_2 and PGI_2 at the atherosclerosis site. Current anti-inflammation treatments that use COX-2 inhibitors indirectly to reduce PGE_2 production may associate with reducing production of the vascular protector and anti-atherosclerosis mediator, PGI_2. To overcome the side effect of COX-2 inhibitors, a specific inhibitor for mPGES-1 would be a better drug to treat vascular inflammation. Thus, targeting mPGES-1 to develop specific anti-inflammation and anti-atherosclerosis drugs becomes a goal of next generation pharmaceutical designs. Elucidation of the different mechanisms of the functional couplings between COX-2 with mPGES-1 and COX-2 with PGIS represent a key step toward the discovery of new drugs for selectively blocking PGE_2 production in inflammation.

EP Receptor Mediated Vascular Inflammation in Atherosclerosis

Molecular cloning has revealed the existence of multiple PGE receptors mediating diverse/opposite biological functions through different signaling pathways via specific G protein couplings [31-34]. PGE_2 binds to EP2 and EP4 receptors acting similarily to the IP receptor by increasing intracellular cAMP through Gs coupling. PGE_2 binds to the EP1 receptor causing an increase in calcium levels similar to the TP receptor through Gq coupling and binds to the EP3 receptor causing a decrease in the cAMP level through Gi coupling [31-34, Figure 2). Development of the subtype-specific EP receptor ligand has been attempted for decades, but not many successful ligands have been discovered thus far. One of the major obstacles is the lack of the 3D structural information describing the molecular mechanism of the specific ligand recognitions in the subtype receptors.

The diverse biological functions of PGE_2 mediated by its isoform receptors were also confirmed by recent gene-knockout experiments [38-39]. Both EP2 and EP4 receptors have been demonstrated to be coupled with the stimulation of cAMP. However, the profiles of gene expression in response to hormones and proinflammatory stimuli have suggested that these two receptors play rather different roles in various physiological processes. It is interesting in this respect to study the phenotypes that appear in the EP2- and EP4- knockout mice. EP2-deficient mice have a slightly impaired ovulation and a dramatic reduction in fertilization. COX-2-deficient mice suffered impaired pregnancies partly due to the dysfunction of the EP2 receptor. In vascular functions, EP2-deficient mice could develop significant hypertension using a high-salt diet. PGE_2 is produced in the body in response to a high-salt diet and works to regulate blood pressure via the relaxant by EP2 receptor [38-39]. However, the fact that EP4 mediates the dilation of ductus artery in the fetus has been confirmed by the gene-knockout experiments. Upon birth, mammals undergo a change from fetal circulation to pulmonary circulation, caused by the closure of the ductus. The ductus in the fetus is principally maintained by the dilation of PGE_2 and PGI_2, and its closure at birth is induced by the withdrawal of PGs as well as by active contraction by increased oxygen tension. Giving indomethacin to mice during late pregnancy indeed induced premature closure of the ductus in wild-type fetuses, but not in the EP4-deficient fetuses, indicating that the dilation of PGE_2 on the vessel is mediated by the EP4 receptor [38-39]. Suppression of PGE_2 by COXs inhibitors in later pregnancy may cause contraction of the ductus and thereby reducing blood circulation for the fetus. In contrast, EP1 and EP3 couple to increase the intracellular Ca2+ mobilization. EP3 is the only prostanoid receptor that inhibits cAMP levels. EP3-knockout in mice failed to show a fever response to pyrogen. EP1-knockout in mice and EP1 antagonist reduced 60% of colon cancer formation [38-39]. The direct relationship of the EP isoforms and vascular inflammation in atherosclerosis in the gene-knockout mice are not well characterized as of yet. However, it is clear that developing subtype inhibitors targeting EP receptors is another possible way to treat vascular inflammation and atherosclerosis in the future.

REFERENCES

[1] Skultetyova, D., Filipova, S., Riecansky, I. and Mistrik, G. (2003) Endothelial dysfunction and the clinical application. *Bratisl. Lek. Listy. 104*, 40-41.

[2] Linton, M.F., Fazio, S. (2002) Cyclooxygenase-2 and atherosclerosis. *Curr. Opin. Lipidol. 13,* 497-504.

[3] Belton, O., Byrne, D., Kearney, D., Leahy, A. and Fitzgerald, D. (2000) Cyclooxygenase-1 and -2-dependent prostacyclin formation in patients with atherosclerosis. *Circulation 102,* 840-845.

[4] Schonbeck, U., Sukhova, G.K., Graber, P., Coulter, S. and Libby, P. (1999) Augmented expression of cyclooxygenase-2 in human atherosclerotic lesions. *Am. J. Pathol. 155*, 1281-1291.

[5] Baker, C.S., Hall, R.J., Evans, T.J., Pomerance, A., Maclouf, J., Creminon, C., Yacoub, M.H. and Polak, J.M. (1999) Cyclooxygenase-2 is widely expressed in atherosclerotic lesions affecting native and transplanted human coronary arteries and colocalizes with inducible nitric oxide synthase and nitrotyrosine particularly in macrophages. Arterioscler. *Thromb. Vasc. Biol. 19*, 646–655.

[6] Fitzgerald, G.A., Pedersen, A.K. and Patrono, C. (1983) Analysis of prostacyclin and thromboxane biosynthesis in cardiovascular disease. *Circulation 67*, 1174-1177.

[7] Massy, Z.A. and Swan, S.K. (2001) Cyclooxygenase-2 and atherosclerosis: friend or foe? Nephrol. *Dial Transplant. 16*, 2286-2289.

[8] Vane, J.R. (2002) Biomedicine. Back to an aspirin a day? *Science 296,* 474-475.

[9] Bombardier, C., Laine, L., Reicin, A., Shapiro, D., Burgos-Vargas, R., Davis, B., Day, R., Ferraz, M.B., Hawkey, C.J., Hochberg, M.C., Kvien, T.K., Schnitzer, T.J. and VIGOR Study Group. (2000) Comparison of upper gastrointestinal toxicity of rofecoxib and naproxen in patients with rheumatoid arthritis. *N. Engl. J. Med. 343*, 1520-1528.

[10] Boers, M. (2001) NSAIDs and selective COX-2 inhibitors: competition between gastroprotection and cardioprotection. *Lancet. 357*, 1222–1223.

[11] Golino, P., Crea, F. and Willerson, J.T. (2002) How to study the effects of platelet aggregation and thrombosis on coronary vasomotion and their clinical relevance. *Ital. Heart J. 3*, 220-225.

[12] Majerus, P.W. (1983) Arachdonate metabolism in vascular disorders. *J. Clin. Invest. 72*, 1521-1525.

[13] Miller, D.K., Sadowski, S., Soderman, D.D. and Kuehl, F.A.Jr. (1985) Endothelial cell prostacyclin production induced by activated neutrophils. *J. Biol. Chem. 260*, 1006-1014.

[14] Smith, W.L. (1986) Prostaglandin biosynthesis and its compartmentation in vascular smooth muscle and endothelial cells. *Annu. Rev. Physiol. 48*, 251-262.

[15] Needleman, P., Turk, J., Jackschik, B.A., Morrison, A.R. and Lefkowith, J.B. (1986) Arachidonic acid metabolism. *Annu. Rev. Biochem. 55*, 69-102.

[16] Granstrom, E., Diczfalusy, U., Hamberg, M., Hansson, G., Malmsten, C. and Samuelson, B. (1982) Prostaglandins and the cardiovascular system (Oates, J.A., ed) pp. 15-58, Raven Press, New York..

[17] Picot, D., Loll, P.J. and Garavitok, R.M. (1994) The X-ray crystal structure of the membrane protein prostaglandin H2 synthase-1. *Nature 367*, 243-249.

[18] Luong, C., Miller, A., Barnett, J., Chow, J., Ramesha, C. and Browner, M.F. (1996) Flexibility of the NSAID binding site in the structure of human cyclooxygenase-2. *Nat. Struct. Biol. 3*, 927-933.

[19] Ohashi, K., Ruan, K.-H., Kulmacz, R.J., Wu, K.K. and Wang, L.-H. (1992) Primary structure of human thromboxane synthase determined from the cDNA sequence. *J. Biol. Chem. 267,* 789-793.

[20] Yokoyama, C., Miyata, A., Ihara, H., Ullrich, V. and Tanabe, T. (1991) Molecular cloning of human platelet thromboxane A synthase. *Biochem. Biophys. Res. Commun. 178*, 1479-1484.

[21] Shen, R.-F., Back, S.J., Zhang, L., Chase, M.B., Tai, H.-H. and Purtell, D.C. (1982) Eighth Int. Conf. on prostaglandins and related compounds. Cloning, expression, and chromosomal mapping thromboxane synthase.

[22] Haurand, M. and Ullrich, V. (1985) Isolation and characterization of thromboxane synthase from human platelets as a cytochrome P450 enzyme. *J. Biol. Chem. 260,* 15059-15067.

[23] Ullrich, V. and Graf, H. (1984) Prostacyclin and thromboxane synthase as P-450 enzymes. *Trends Pharmacol. Sci. 5*, 352-355.

[24] Ravichandran, K. G., Boddupalli, S. S., Hasemann, C. A., Peterson, J. A., and Deisenhofer, J. (1993) Crystal structure of hemoprotein domain of P450BM-3, a prototype for microsomal P450's. *Science 261,* 731-736.

[25] Ruan, K.-H., Milfeld, K., Kulmacz, R.J. and Wu K.K. (1994) Comparison of the construction of a 3-D model for human thromboxane synthase using P450cam and BM-3 as templates: implications for the substrate binding pocket. *Protein Eng. 7,* 1345-1351.

[26] Wang, L.-H., Matijevic-Aleksic, N., Hsu, P.Y., Ruan, K.-H., Wu, K.K. and Kulmacz, R.J. (1996) Identification of thromboxane A_2 synthase active site residues by molecular modeling-guided site-directed mutagenesis. *J. Biol. Chem. 33*, 19970-19975.

[27] Ushikubi, F., Nakajima, M., Hirata, M., Okuma, M., Fujiwara, M. and Narumiya, S. (1989) Purification of the thromboxane A_2/prostagiandin H_2, receptor from human blood platelets. *J. Biol. Chem. 264*, 16496-16501.

[28] Hirata, M., Hayashi, Y., Ushikubi, F., Yokata, Y., Kageyama, R., Nakanishi, S., and Narumiya, S. (1991) Cloning and expression of cDNA for a human thromboxane A_2, receptor. *Nature 349,* 617-620.

[29] Katsuyama, M., Sugimoto, Y., Namba, T., Irie, A., Negishi, M., Narumiya, S. and Ichikawa, A. (1994) Cloning and expression of a cDNA for the human prostacyclin receptor. *FEBS Lett. 344*, 74-88.

[30] Abrarnovitz, M., Boie, Y., Nguyen, T., Rushmore, T.H., Bayne, M.A., Metters, K.M., Slipetz, D.M. and Grygorczyk, R. (1994) Cloning and expression of a cDNA for tile human prostanoid FP receptor. *J. Biol. Chem. 269,* 1356-1360.

[31] Funk, C.D., Furci, L., FitzGerald, G.A., Grygorczyk, R., Rochette, C., Bayne, M.A., Abramovitz, M., Adam, M. and Metters, K.M. (1993) Cloning and expression of

CDNA for the human prostaglandin E receptor EP1 subtype. *J. Biol. Chem. 268*, 26767-26772.

[32] An, S., Yang, J., Xia, M. and Goetzl, E.J. (1993) Cloning and expression of the EP2 subtype of human receptors for prostaglandin E_2. Biochem. *Biophys. Res. Commun. 197*, 263-270.

[33] Bastien, L., Sawyer, N., Grygorczyk, R., Metters, M. and Adam, M. (1994) Alternative splicing produces a divergent cytoplasmic tail in the human endothelial thromboxane A_2, receptor. *J. Biol. Chem. 269*, 11873-11877.

[34] Adam, M., Boie, Y., Rushmore, T.H., Muller, G., Bastien, L., McKee, K.T., Metters, K. M. and Abramovitz, M. (1994) Cloning and expression of three isoforms of the human EP_3 prostanoid receptor. *FEBS Lett. 338*, 170-174.

[35] Regan, J.W., Bailey, T.J., Donello, J.E., Pierce, K.L., Pepperi, D.J., Zhang, D., Kedzie, K.M., Fairbaim, C.D., Bogardus, A.M., Woodward, D.F. and Gil, D.W. (1994) Molecular cloning and expression of human EP_3 receptors: evidence of three variants with differing carboxyl termini. *Br. J. Pharmacol. 112*, 377-385.

[36] Kunapuli, S.P., Mao, G.F., Bastepe, M., Liu-Chen, L.Y., Li, S., Cheung, P.P., DeRiel, J.K. and Ashby, B. (1994) Cloning and expression of a prostaglandin E receptor EP_3 subtype from human erythroleukaemia cells. *Biochem. J.* 298, 263-267.

[37] Yang, J., Xia, M., Goetzl, E. J. and An, S. (1994) Cloning and expression of the EP_3-subtype of human receptors for prostaglandin E_2. Biochem. *Biophys. Res. Commun. 198*, 999-1006.

[38] Kobayashi T, Narumiya S. (2002) Function of prostanoid receptors: studies on knockout mice. *Prostaglandins Other Lipid Mediat. 68-69*, 557-573.

[39] Narumiya, S. and FitzGerald, G.A. (2001) Genetic and pharmacological analysis of prostanoid receptor function. *J. Clin. Invest. 108*, 25-30.

[40] Sugimoto, Y., Narumiya, S. and Ichikawa A. (2000) Distribution and function of prostanoid receptors: studies from knockout mice. *Prog. Lipid Res. 39*, 289-314.

[41] Thomas, D.W., Mannon, R.B., Mannon, P.J., Latour, A., Oliver, J.A., Hoffman, M., Smithies, O., Koller, B.H. and Coffman, T.M. (1998) Coagulation defects and altered hemodynamic responses in mice lacking receptors for thromboxane A2. *J. Clin. Invest. 102*, 1994-2001.

[42] Negishi, M., Sugimoto, Y. and Ichikawa, A. (1995) Molecular mechanisms of diverse actions of prostanoid receptors. Biochim. *Biophys. Acta 1259*, 109-120.

[43] Funk, C.D., Furci, L., Moran, N., and Fitzgerald, G.A. (1993) Point mutation in the seventh hydrophobic domain of the human thromboxane A_2 receptor allows discrimination between agonist and antagonist binding sites. *Mol. Pharmacol. 44*, 934-939.

[44] Yamamoto, Y., Kamiya, K. and Terao, S. (1993) Modeling of human thromboxane A_2 receptor and analysis of the receptor-ligand interaction. *J. Med. Chem. 36*, 820-825.

[45] Chiang, N., Kan, W.M. and Tai, H.H. (1996) Site-directed mutagenesis of cysteinyl and serine residues of human thromboxane A_2 receptor in insect cells. *Arch. Biochem. Biophys. 334*, 9-17.

[46] Breyer, R.M and Audoly, L. (1997) The second extracellular loop of the prostaglandin EP3 receptor is an essential determinant of ligand selectivity. *J. Biol. Chem. 272*, 13475-13478.

[47] Turek, J.W., Halmos, T., Sullivan, N.L., Antonakis, K. and Le Breton, G.C. (2002) Mapping of a ligand-binding site for the human thromboxane A_2 receptor protein. *J. Biol. Chem. 277*, 16791-16797.

[48] So, S.-P., Wu, J., Huang, G., Huang, A., Li, D. and Ruan, K.-H. (2003) Identification of residues important for ligand binding of thromboxane A_2 receptor in the second extracellular loop using the NMR experiment-guided mutagenesis approach. *J. Biol. Chem. 278,* 10922-10927.

[49] Henderson, R., Baldwin, J.M., Ceska, T.A., Zemlin, F., Beckmann, E. and Downing, K.H. (1990) Model for the structure of bacteriorhodopsin based on high-resolution electron cryo-microscopy. *J. Mol. Biol. 213*, 899-929.

[50] Grigorieff, N., Ceska, T.A., Downing, K.H., Baldwin, J.M. and Henderson, R. (1996) Electron-crystallographic refinement of the structure of bacteriorhodopsin. *J. Mol. Biol. 259*, 393-421.

[51] Pebay-Peyroula, E., Rummell, G., Rosenbusch, J.P. and Landau, E.M. (1997) X-ray structure of bacteriorhodopsin at 2.5 angstroms from microcrystals grown in lipidic cubic phases. *Science 277*, 1676-1681.

[52] Palczewski, K., Kumasaka, T., Hori, T., Behnke, C.A., Motoshima, H., Fox, B.A., Le Trong, I., Teller, D.C., Okada, T., Stenkamp, R.E., Yamamoto, M. and Miyano, M. (2000) Crystal structure of rhodopsin: A G protein-coupled receptor. *Science 289*, 739-745.

[53] Ruan, K.-H., So, S.-P., Wu, J., Li, D., Huang, A. and Kung, J. (2001) Solution structure of the second extracellular loop of human thromboxane A_2 receptor. *Biochemistry 40*, 275-280.

[54] Wu, J., So, S.-P. and Ruan, K.-H. (2003) Solution structure of the third extracellular loop of human thromboxane A_2 receptor. Arch. Biochem. *Biophys*. 414, 287-293.

[55] Dorn, G.W.2nd (1990) Cyclic oxidation-reduction reactions regulate thromboxane A_2/prostaglandin H_2 receptor number and affinity in human platelet membranes. J. Biol. *Chem*. *265,* 4240-4246.

[56] D'Angelo, D.D., Eubank, J.J., Davis, M.G. and Dorn, G.W.2nd. (1996) Mutagenic analysis of platelet thromboxane receptor cysteines. *J. Biol. Chem. 271*, 6233-6240.

[57] Mayeux, P.R., Morinelli, T.A., Williams, T.C., Hazard, E.S., Mais, D.E., Oatis, J.E., Baron, D.A. and Halushka, P.V. (1991) Differential effect of pH on thromboxane A_2/prostaglandin H_2 receptor agonist and antagonist binding in human platelets. *J. Biol. Chem. 266*, 13752-13758.

[58] Dorn, G.W.2nd, Davis, M.G. and D'Angelo, D.D. (1997) Structural determinants for agonist binding affinity to thromboxane/prostaglandin endoperoxide (TP) receptors. Analysis of chimeric rat/human TP receptors. *J. Biol. Chem. 272*, 12399-12405.

[59] Dogne, J.M., de Leval, X., Delarge, J., David, J.L. and Masereel, B. (2000) New trends in thromboxane and prostacyclin modulators. *Curr. Med. Chem. 7*, 609-628.

[60] Von Baeyer, H., Hopfenmuller, W., Riedel, E. and Affeld, K. (2003) Atherosclerosis: current concepts of pathophysiology and pharmacological intervention based on trial outcomes. *Clin. Nephrol. 60 (Suppl 1)*, 31-48.

[61] McAdam, B.F., Catella-Lawson, F., Mardini, I.A., Kapoor, S., Lawson, J.A. and FitzGerald, G.A. (1999) Systemic biosynthesis of prostacyclin by cyclooxygenase (COX)-2: the human pharmacology of a selective inhibitor of COX-2. *Proc. Natl. Acad. Sci. USA 96,* 272–277.

[62] Reis, E.D., Roque, M., Dansky, H., Fallon, J.T., Badimon, J.J., Cordon-Cardo, C., Shiff, S.J. and Fisher, E.A. (2000) Sulindac inhibits neointimal formation after arterial injury in wild-type and apolipoprotein E-deficient mice. *Proc. Natl. Acad. Sci. USA 97*, 12764-12769.

[63] Pratico, D., Tillmann, C., Zhi-Bing, Z., Hongwei, L. and FitzGerald, G.A. (2001) Acceleration of atherogenesis by COX-1-dependent prostanoid formation in low density lipoprotein receptor knockout mice. *Proc. Natl. Acad. Sci. USA 98*, 3358-3363.

[64] Kvasnicka, T., (2003) NO (nitric oxide) and its significance in regulation of vascular homeostasis. *Vnitr. Lek. 49*, 291-296.

[65] Arbab, F., Goldsby, J., Matijevic-Aleksic, N., Huang, G., Ruan, K.H. and Huang, J.C. (2002) Prostacyclin is an autocrine regulator in the contraction of oviductal smooth muscle. *Hum. Reprod. 17*, 3053-3059.

[66] Huang, J.C., Arbab, F., Tumbusch, K.J., Goldsby, J.S., Matijevic-Aleksic, N. and Wu, K.K. (2002) Human fallopian tubes express prostacyclin (PGI) synthase and cyclooxygenases and synthesize abundant PGI. *J. Clin. Endocrinol. Metab. 87*, 4361-4368.

[67] Debey, S., Meyer-Kirchrath, J. and Schror, K. (2003) Regulation of cyclooxygenase-2 expression by iloprost in human vascular smooth muscle cells. Role of transcription factors CREB and ICER. Biochem. *Pharmacol. 65*, 979-988.

[68] Ruan, K.-H., So, S.-P., Zheng, W., Wu, J., Li, D. and Kung, J. (2002) Solution structure and topology of the N-terminal membrane anchor domain of a microsomal cytochrome P450: prostaglandin I_2 synthase. *Biochem. J.* 368, 1-7.

[69] Lin, Y.Z., Deng, H. and Ruan, K.-H. (2000) Topology of catalytic portion of prostaglandin I(2) synthase: identification by molecular modeling-guided site-specific antibodies. *Arch. Biochem. Biophys. 379*, 188-197.

[70] Deng, H., Huang, A., So, S.P., Lin, Y.Z. and Ruan, K.-H. (2002) Substrate access channel topology in membrane-bound prostacyclin synthase. *Biochem. J. 362*, 545-551.

[71] Boie, Y., Rushmore, T.H., Darmon-Goodwin, A., Grygorczyk, R., Slipetz, D.M., Metters, K.M. and Abramovitz, M.J. (1994) Cloning and expression of a cDNA for the human prostanoid IP receptor. *J. Biol. Chem. 269*, 12173-12178.

[72] Nakagawa, O., Tanaka, I., Usui, T., Harada, M., Sasaki, Y., Itoh, H., Yoshimasa, T., Namba, T., Narumiya, S. and Nakao, K. (1994) Molecular cloning of human prostacyclin receptor cDNA and its gene expression in the cardiovascular system. *Circulation 90*, 1643-1647.

[73] Kaliman, J., Sinzinger, H., Staudacher, M. and Mannheimer, E. (1985) Defects in the prostaglandin system. II. Familial platelet-prostacyclin receptor defect (Wien-Hietzing

defect)--pathogenetic significance for (early) development of atherosclerosis? *Wien Klin Wochenschr 97*, 323-326.

[74] Watanabe, Y., Matsumura, K., Takechi, H., Kato, K., Morii, H., Bjorkman, M., Langstrom, B., Noyori, R., Suzuki, M. and Watanabe, Y. (1999) A novel subtype of prostacyclin receptor in the central nervous system. *J. Neurochem. 72*, 2583-2592.

[75] Issemann, I. and Green, S. (1990) Activation of a member of the steroid hormone receptor superfamily by peroxisome proliferators. *Nature 347*, 645-650.

[76] Zhang, J., Fu, M., Zhu, X., Xiao, Y., Mou, Y., Zheng, H., Akinbami, M.A., Wang, Q. and Chen, Y.E. (2002) Peroxisome proliferator-activated receptor delta is up-regulated during vascular lesion formation and promotes post-confluent cell proliferation in vascular smooth muscle cells. *J. Biol. Chem. 277*, 11505-11512.

[77] Plutzky, J. (2003) Medicine. PPARs as therapeutic targets: reverse cardiology? *Science 302*, 406-407.

[78] Ouchi, N., Kihara, S., Funahashi, T., Matsuzawa, Y. and Walsh, K. (2003) Obesity, adiponectin and vascular inflammatory disease. *Curr. Opin. Lipidol. 14*, 561-566.

[79] Gonzalez, M.A., and Selwyn, A.P. (2003) Endothelial function, inflammation, and prognosis in cardiovascular disease. *Am. J. Med. 115 Suppl 8A*, 99S-106S.

[80] Murakami, M., Nakatani, Y., Tanioka, T. and Kudo, I. (2002) Prostaglandin E synthase. *Prostaglandins Other Lipid Mediat. 68-69*, 383-399.

[81] Tanioka, T., Nakatani, Y., Semmyo, N., Murakami, M. and Kudo, I. (2000) Molecular identification of cytosolic prostaglandin E2 synthase that is functionally coupled with cyclooxygenase-1 in immediate prostaglandin E2 biosynthesis. *J. Biol. Chem. 275*, 32775-32782.

[82] Murakami, M., Nakashima, K., Kamei, D., Masuda, S., Ishikawa, Y., Ishii, T., Ohmiya, Y., Watanabe, K. and Kudo, I. (2003) Cellular prostaglandin E2 production by membrane-bound prostaglandin E synthase-2 via both cyclooxygenases-1 and -2. *J. Biol. Chem. 278*, 37937-37947.

[83] Cipollone, F., Prontera, C., Pini, B., Marini, M., Fazia, M., De Cesare, D., Iezzi, A., Ucchino, S., Boccoli, G., Saba, V., Chiarelli, F., Cuccurullo, F., Mezzetti, A. (2001) Overexpression of functionally coupled cyclooxygenase-2 and prostaglandin E synthase in symptomatic atherosclerotic plaques as a basis of prostaglandin E(2)-dependent plaque instability. *Circulation 104*, 921-927.

ACKNOWLEDGEMENTS

I thank Lori Jenkins and Shui-Ping So for the assistance of the manuscript preparation.

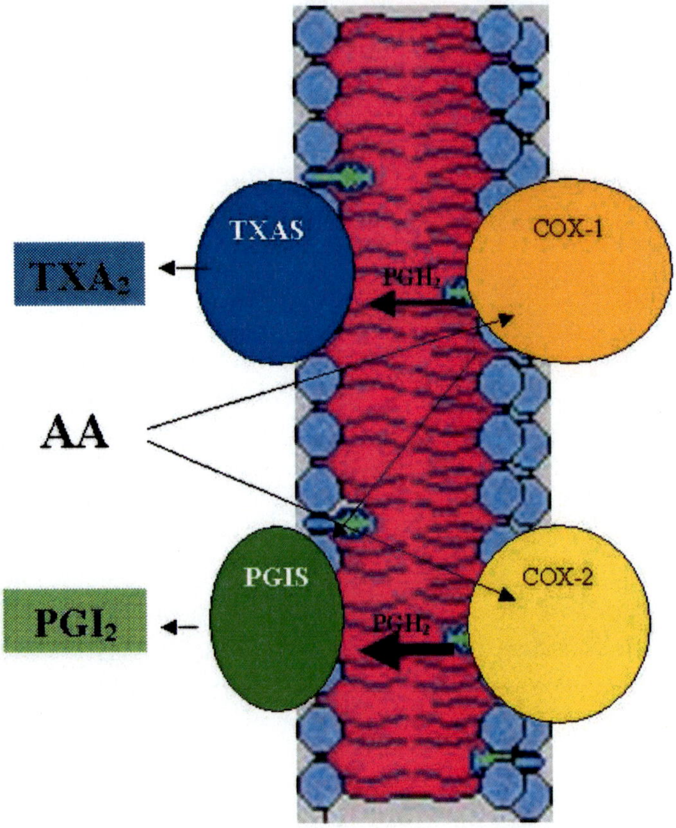

Figure 3. Membrane topological models of the COXs, TXAS and PGIS, and the biosynthesis of TXA_2 and PGI_2 in the ER membrane.

In: Current Topics in Atherosclerosis Research
Editor: Yong J. Geng, pp. 103-132

ISBN 1-59454-428-X

Chapter VI

Atherosclerosis in Patients with Chronic Kidney Disease

Diana I. Jalal, and Bruce C. Kone***

Division of Renal Diseases and Hypertension, Department of Internal Medicine, The University of Texas Health Science Center at Houston, School of Medicine

Abstract

Cardiovascular disease (CVD) stands out as the major contributor to the increased mortality in patients with chronic kidney disease (CKD). In this chapter, we shed light on the reported increased incidence of atherosclerosis in this group of patients, as well as on the various risk factors that have been implicated in association with this pathological process. While the traditional risk factors that are associated with an increased risk of atherosclerotic CVD in the general population are quite prevalent in patients with underlying CKD, they do not appear to account solely for the increased risk in this particular group of patients. Furthermore, certain differences exist in the relationship between some of these factors and CVD in this patient population. We also explore in greater detail the "non-traditional" risk factors, such as systemic inflammation, oxidative and carbonyl stress, malnutrition, and abnormal calcium and phosphorus metabolism, and their potential accentuated contribution to the atherosclerotic process in CKD patients. Some of these non-traditional risk factors stand as appealing therapeutic targets that might help modulate the progression of atherosclerosis in these patients.

Keywords: Vascular disease, renal failure, inflammation, oxidative stress.

---

* Correspondence concerning this article should be addressed to Dr. Bruce C. Kone, M.D., FACP, FCP, FAHA, FASN, Division of Renal Diseases and Hypertension The University of Texas Medical School at Houston, 6431 Fannin, MSB 4.138. Houston, TX 77030.

INTRODUCTION

Over 25 years ago, Lindner et al. [68] noted the increasing role of cardiovascular disease in the mortality of patients with stage 5 chronic kidney disease (CKD)[1]: "as patients' survival has approached the 10 year mark, there has been an increasing indication that accelerated atherosclerosis may become the major unresolved problem threatening the longevity of patients on regular hemodialysis." It is now acknowledged that cardiovascular disease is the most common contributor to the mortality of patients with CKD. The prevalence of coronary artery disease in stage 5 CKD patients on maintenance dialysis is estimated to be about 40% [35]. Even after stratification for age, gender and the presence or absence of diabetes, patients with CKD remain at a 10 to 20 times higher risk of death from cardiovascular disease. Half of the deaths in the Hypertension Detection and Follow-up Program (HDFP) study involving nearly 11,000 participants (16% diabetic) occurred in individuals with baseline serum creatinines of >1.7 mg/dL [116]. In the British Regional Heart Study of 7690 men (<2 % diabetic) followed for more than 14 years, cardiovascular causes accounted for more than half of all deaths in subjects within the upper decile of baseline serum creatinine [139]. Even patients with mild renal impairment suffer from increased risk for clinically significant coronary artery disease and stroke. The fact that CKD patients appear to have accelerated atherosclerosis is of particular public health importance given the exploding incidence of CKD both in the United States and worldwide. Just as worrisome, the true incidence and prevalence of atherosclerosis in CKD patients may be underestimated [126].

Patients with CKD suffer from at least two subtypes of arterial vascular disease: atherosclerosis and large-vessel remodeling or arteriosclerosis [72]. Studies focused on atherosclerosis, such as those measuring carotid artery intima-media thickness (CA-IMT) or evaluating myocardial infarction or stroke in patients with CKD, confirm that patients with CKD suffer from a higher incidence of atherosclerotic complications, and suggest that the atherosclerotic process starts before the onset of chronic dialysis [47,70]. It remains unclear why patients with CKD suffer from an accelerated process of atherosclerosis. It is felt, however, that the risk factors traditionally associated with atherosclerosis, namely age, gender, smoking, hyperlipidemia and diabetes, are insufficient to account for the extent and the severity of cardiovascular complications in this patient population [102]. Consequently, other factors specific to CKD may also promote cardiovascular disease among CKD patients.

This chapter focuses on the clinical and experimental basis for accelerated atherosclerosis in CKD patients and analyzes conventional and novel therapeutic interventions that may improve cardiovascular outcome in these patients. While it is recognized that diabetes mellitus is an important contributor to the development of both CKD and atherosclerosis and that the kidney transplant patient commonly suffers from atherosclerotic disease, this chapter will not specifically address these clinical settings.

---

[1] Stage 5 chronic kidney disease is equivalent to end-stage kidney disease according to the new NKF-K/DOQI™ classification scheme (see Table 1 for explanation of stages).

Table 1. Classification of Chronic Kidney Disease

CKD Stage	Description	GFR (ml/min/1.73m^2)	U.S. prevalence, %
1	Kidney damage with normal or ↑ GFR	≥ 90	3.3
2	Kidney damage with mild ↓in GFR	60-89	3.0
3	Moderate ↓ in GFR	30-59	4.3
4	Severe ↓ in GFR	15-29	0.2
5	Kidney failure	≤ 15 or dialysis	0.1

From the "Kidney Disease Outcomes Quality Initiative Clinical Practice Guidelines for Chronic Kidney Disease: Evaluation, Classification and Stratification." Adapted with permission from the National Kidney Foundation. Abbreviations: CKD, chronic kidney disease; GFR, glomerular filtration rate.

CHRONIC KIDNEY DISEASE

According to a recently developed consensus statement, the National Kidney Foundation defines CKD by the presence of kidney damage and clinically stages the disease by the level of kidney function. In this schema, there are five stages of progressive severity of kidney dysfunction, the most advanced of which, stage 5, is end-stage kidney disease requiring renal replacement therapy in the form of dialysis or kidney transplantation (Table 1). It should be noted that stage 1 CKD includes patients with evidence of kidney damage despite normal or even elevated glomerular filtration rate (GFR). For example, patients with albuminuria may have substantial kidney damage, yet have relatively preserved GFR of greater than 60 ml/min/1.73m^2. These patients are included in the staging system, because they are at increased risk of the two major outcomes of CKD --- loss of kidney function and the development of cardiovascular complications.

CHRONIC KIDNEY DISEASE AND ATHEROSCLEROSIS

Recent clinical and autopsy studies in pre-dialysis and dialysis cohorts have demonstrated that atherosclerotic lesions in kidney failure are frequently calcified (principally containing hydroxylapatite), rather than fibroatheromatous, have increased media thickness of the intima and media, and are more highly infiltrated with activated macrophages compared with lesions in the general population. The increased intima and media thickness develops early in the course of CKD, and appears to be modified at least in part by parathyroid hormone (PTH) and endothelin-1 (ET-1), both of which are elevated in patients with CKD [105]. In animal models of kidney failure, a direct effect of high phosphorus diet in mediating arterial wall thickening was also documented. The calcifications in stage 5 CKD patients may limit the utility of electron-beam computed tomography as a sensitive method to detect atherosclerosis, because it is unable to distinguish between intimal calcifications of atherosclerosis and the medial calcification common in stage 5 CKD.

Recent studies have established that microalbuminuria is an indicator of endothelial dysfunction and predicts cardiovascular mortality in patients with diabetes and/or hypertension [50, 79, 87, 88, 109]. A few studies have demonstrated an association between microalbuminuria and increased CA-IMT in patients with primary hypertension [66,95], whereas one study analyzing microalbuminuria and CA-IMT in otherwise healthy subjects failed to demonstrate such an association [4]. The available evidence suggests that in patients with hypertension and diabetes, microalbuminuria is indeed the end-result of a pathological process leading to endothelial injury and plaque formation. Although it would be difficult to argue that CKD at this early stage is responsible for accelerating the atherosclerotic process, it does appear that atherosclerosis is advanced in patients with later stages of CKD but not yet requiring dialysis. For example, Shoji et al. [113] have shown increased CA-IMT in non-diabetic patients with CKD prior to onset of dialysis, as compared to healthy control subjects. Another study focused specifically on atherosclerotic cardiovascular disease outcomes and assessed the incidence of myocardial and cerebral infarction in 748 patients before or after initiation of chronic dialysis. The incidence of myocardial infarction was approximately 2-3 times higher in the CKD patients as compared to the general population and did not differ between the pre- and post-dialysis groups, suggesting that factors related to CKD rather than dialysis itself are responsible for this increased risk [53]. It remains to be established, however, whether there is a threshold level of GFR below which cardiovascular disease risk accelerates in a nonlinear fashion.

Traditional Cardiovascular Risk Factors and Chronic Kidney Disease

Though the cardiovascular risk conferred to CKD patients by traditional risk factors generally mirrors that of the general population, some risk factors for developing symptomatic ischemic heart disease may be more prevalent in patients with CKD compared to the general population (Table 2). Data from the National Health and Nutrition Examination Survey (NHANES) III show an inverse association between older age and reduced GFR, and a much higher prevalence of diabetes and hypertension in subjects with elevated serum creatinine levels (1.6 mg/dL in men and 1.4 mg/dL in women) [22]. Although, the cardiovascular risk conferred to CKD patients by such traditional risk factors as diabetes, older age, and left ventricular hypertrophy, generally mirrors that of the general population, some important differences exist. For example, U-shaped relationships exist between all-cause mortality and both cholesterol levels and blood pressure in stage 5 CKD patients, likely reflecting the confounding effects, respectively, of malnutrition [102] and cardiomyopathy. Moreover, most studies have failed to demonstrate a clear association between serum lipids and cardiovascular disease in ESKD patients. Some traditional risk factors also appear to be shared risk factors for the development of cardiovascular disease and CKD. For example, hypertension increases the risk of both ischemic heart disease and CKD. Accordingly, the seventh report of the Joint National Committee for the Prevention, Detection, Evaluation and

Treatment of High Blood Pressure (JNC-7) includes CKD as a "compelling" indication for medical treatment and prescribes both a lower target blood pressure and treatment with specific antihypertensive agents compared to the general population [21].

Table 2. Traditional and Chronic Kidney Disease-related Risk Factors for Cardiovascular Disease

Traditional Cardiovascular Disease Risk Factors	CKD-related (Nontraditional) Cardiovascular Disease Risk Factors
Older age	Albuminuria
Male gender	Volume overload; sustained and refractory hypertension
White race	Abnormal calcium and phosphorus metabolism, vascular calcification
Hypertension	Malnutrition
↑ LDL cholesterol	Chronic anemia
↓ HDL cholesterol	Systemic inflammation
Diabetes mellitus	↑ oxidative stress
Smoking	Altered lipoprotein(a), apolipoprotein(a) metabolism
Physical inactivity	Hyperhomocysteinemia
Psychosocial stress	Altered balance of vasoactive molecules (nitric oxide/endothelin)
Family history of cardiovascular disease	
Left ventricular hypertrophy	

CKD - chronic kidney disease.

Uremic patients exhibit a complex dyslipidemia involving defective lipoprotein uptake and metabolism [17]. The most prominent finding is an increase in triglycerides without an increase in total cholesterol. Intermediate-density lipoprotein (IDL) and very low density lipoprotein (VLDL) levels, however, are elevated [115,140]. Shoji et al. [114] demonstrated that IDL is the lipoprotein fraction most closely associated with abnormal aortic pulse wave velocity, used as an indicator of atherosclerosis. These authors proposed that IDL should be the lipoprotein fraction targeted in the management of uremic dyslipidemia; however no clinical guidelines exist on achieving appropriate target levels of IDL.

Several studies have labeled lipoprotein(a) [Lp(a)] as an independent risk factor for coronary artery disease in the general population [15, 98, 117]. Cressman et al. [23] reported that Lp(a) levels greater than 38.4 mg/dl predicted adverse cardiovascular events in a cohort of 129 hemodialysis patients. More recently, Ohkuma et al. [90] reported elevated levels of Lp(a) in 59 patients on peritoneal dialysis, and correlated these elevated levels with carotid atherosclerosis. Many studies in the non-uremic population have shown apolipoprotein (apo) E to modulate lipid metabolism, and that the expression of the E4 allele is related to hyperlipidemia and atherosclerosis [56, 86, 141]. The relationship between apo E polymorphism and atherosclerosis in stage 5 CKD patients has been investigated in a few small studies. Guz et al. [41] found no statistically significant relationship between apo E4 polymorphism and CA-IMT in 269 hemodialysis patients. Thus, the atherogenic role of uremic dyslipidemia remains unclear, and the effect of specific lipid-lowering therapies on cardiovascular mortality in CKD patients remains to be determined. However, the recently published "NKF-K/DOQI Clinical Practice Guidelines on Managing Dyslipidemia in Chronic Kidney Disease" recommend that all patients with CKD be included in the highest-risk group, and thus have a lower low-density lipoprotein cholesterol level targeted [2].

Non-traditional Risk Factors

Other factors more apparent in CKD, such as systemic inflammation, increased oxidative and carbonyl stress, impaired nitric oxide bioavailability, hyperhomocysteinemia, chronic anemia, elevated serum phosphate and associated vascular calcification, also promote cardiovascular disease among these patients (Table 2). However, there are no intervention trials from patients with CKD demonstrating that the modification of these non-traditional risk factors reduces CVD.

Systemic Inflammation

It is now acknowledged that systemic inflammation plays an important role in the atherosclerotic process in non-CKD patients by contributing to endothelial cell injury and further plaque formation [99]. In the Physicians Health Study, C-reactive protein (CRP) level was found to be an independent predictor of myocardial infarction and stroke. It was also noted that the reduction in the risk of myocardial infarction seen with the use of aspirin was directly related to the level of CRP [57, 91, 92, 96, 97, 118]. Elevated levels of CRP and interleukin-6 (IL-6) have been demonstrated in patients with CKD in the dialysis as well as the pre-dialysis stages [106, 118, 120, 124, 147]. In a study of 280 stable hemodialysis patients, a stepwise increase in all-cause and cardiovascular mortality rate with increasing quartiles of C-reactive protein (CRP) was observed [144]. Patients with CRP levels in the highest quartile suffered nearly a 5-fold increase in all-cause and cardiovascular mortality compared with patients with the lowest CRP levels, an effect that was independent of several other known mortality predictors.

Since injections with IL-6 exacerbate atherogenesis in mice [48], it has been proposed that this cytokine is more than a mere marker of the atherosclerotic process but may actually contribute to early lesion development [48] (Figure 1). IL-6 levels have been shown to correlate with acute myocardial infarction in the general population. In stage 5 CKD patients, an elevated IL-6 level is not only a predictor of increased mortality, but is also independently associated with carotid atherosclerosis [120,124]. Increased serum levels of IL-18 have also been shown to predict fatal and non-fatal cardiovascular events [11,12]. Conversely, IL-10, an anti-inflammatory cytokine, seems to be protective against coronary events in the general population [19] as well as in stage 5 CKD patients [38]. Indeed, IL-10 deficient mice are more prone to atherosclerosis [77]. Girndt et al. [39] recently discovered that stage 5 CKD patients with the "high-producer" genotype of IL-10 had a lower cardiac event rate and event mortality than the "low-producer" genotype of IL-10. It remains plausible that the balance between pro- and anti-inflammatory cytokines is more important than their actual levels in predicting cardiovascular mortality.

Platelets and platelet-leukocyte aggregates are now known to contribute to ongoing injury at atheromatous sites and in plaque disruption. Ashman et al. [7] luated 48 non-diabetic patients without coronary artery disease but with stage 5 CKD on hemodialysis or chronic ambulatory peritoneal dialysis (CAPD) and demonstrated increased platelet-monocyte aggregates in both patient groups; this finding was associated with an increased risk of cardiovascular disease (Figure 1). Their results may suggest yet another mechanism by which atherosclerosis ensues is such patients. While it is likely that inflammation plays an important role in accelerated atherosclerosis in stage 5 CKD patients, the exact role of these inflammatory markers remains undefined, and it is also unclear whether their pro-atherogenic effect is exerted via direct or indirect participation in lesion formation.

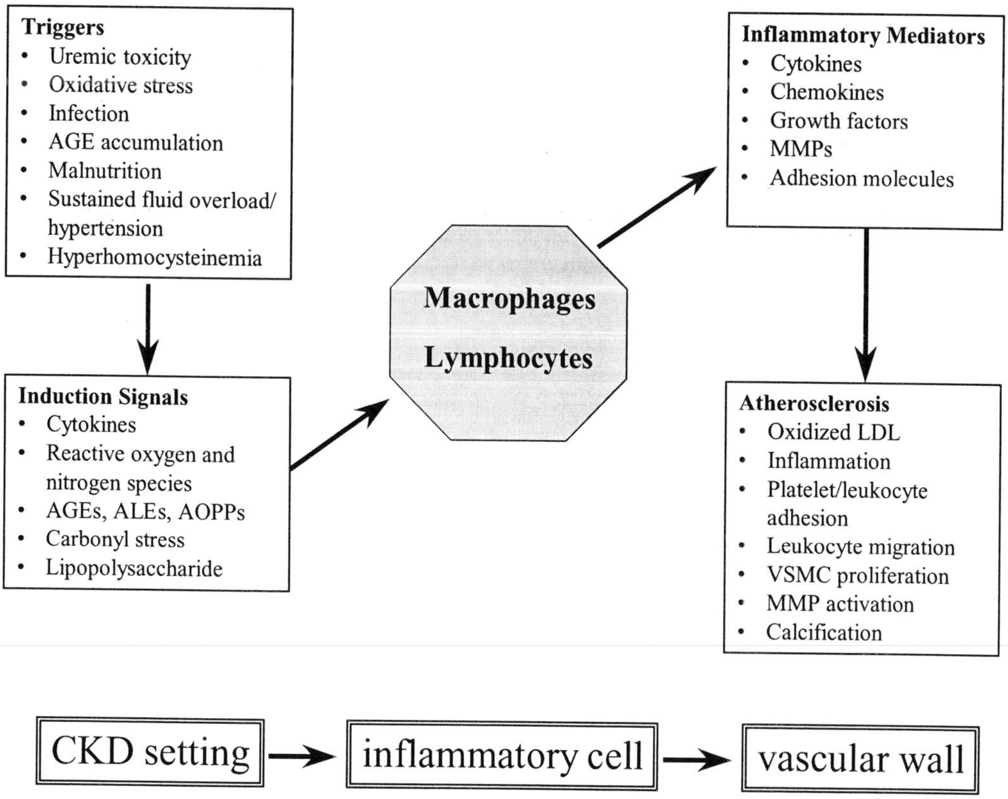

Figure 1. Pivotal role of inflammatory cells in the pathogenesis of atherosclerosis in chronic kidney disease patients. Pathologic circumstances in chronic kidney disease activate induction signals, such as reactive oxygen species, advanced glycation end-products (AGE), advanced lipoxidation end-products (ALEs), and advanced oxidative protein products (AOPPs), that trigger inflammatory cells to transcribe a number of proinflammatory genes. These inflammatory mediators collectively act to accelerate atherogenesis, through oxidation of LDL, leukocyte recruitment and adhesion, vascular smooth muscle cell (VSMC) proliferation, vascular calcification, and matrix metalloproteinase (MMP) activation.

Oxidative Stress

Oxidant-derived tissue injury takes place when the production of oxidants exceeds the local antioxidant capacity. The generation of oxidative compounds is physiologically important as a step in inflammation and tissue repair processes. However when improper activation of the oxidative processes occurs, cell and tissue injury may occur. For example, increased production of reactive oxygen species (ROS) in the vascular wall is evident in and characteristic of atherosclerosis [18,126] (Figure 1). Mitochondria are the most powerful cellular source of ROS, but relatively little is known about their contribution to cellular pathology by this mechanism. The phagocyte oxidant generation system utilizes high levels of oxygen and several enzymes, such as superoxide dismutase, NADPH-oxidase, nitric oxide synthase (NOS), and myeloperoxidase (MPO) to produce reactive oxygen and nitrogen intermediates to aid in the destruction of pathological microorganisms. Increased oxidative stress can lead to oxidation of important macromolecules including proteins, lipids, carbohydrates and DNA. These ROS are produced in small quantities, and they are highly reactive in vivo, so that direct detection of them is extremely difficult. Thus stable end-products of oxidation --- advanced lipoxidation end-products (ALEs), advanced oxidative protein products (AOPPs), and advanced glycation products (AGEs) --- have been exploited as biochemical markers to measure indirectly oxidative stress [6] (Figure1).

CKD appears to be a disease characterized by markedly increased oxidation and impaired antioxidant systems. The increased oxidative stress and reduced capacity to handle oxidative stress is evident prior to dialysis initiation and further exacerbated by it [51, 74, 125]. Recent results also suggest that inflammation interacts with oxidative stress in CKD patients. One study designed to evaluate oxidative stress in stage 5 CKD compared 15 patients with CKD prior to initiation of hemodialysis, 15 patients with stage 5 CKD on maintenance hemodialysis, and 15 healthy controls. Malondialdehyde, a lipid-derived biomarker of oxidative stress, was elevated in dialysis patients compared to CKD and control subjects. Moreover, the antioxidants vitamin C, selenium and glutathione peroxidase were decreased in dialysis patients and, to a lesser extent, in the CKD group compared to the control subjects [74]. Although dialytic therapy improves the redox balance, other factors related to dialysis, such as recurrent infections may contribute to increased oxidative stress [121, 123].

Iatrogenic factors may also contribute to oxidative stress in chronic dialysis patients. For example, intravenous iron, commonly used to replete iron stores in the management of anemia of CKD, may lead to oxidant stress and accelerated atherosclerosis. When iron is administered to the extent that it overwhelms the capacity of carrier proteins, the resultant free iron may be taken up by a variety of tissues with potential production of ROS. Heme, an abundant source of redox-active iron once released from the intracellular heme-containing proteins, can potentiate cytotoxicity by polymorphonuclear leukocytes, and can promote conversion of LDL to its cytotoxic oxidized products, enhancing endothelial cell damage [9]. In a recent study, 17 hemodialysis patients were infused ferric gluconate in single doses of 62.5 mg or 125 mg, or no iron during the first hour of dialysis. The 125 mg dose caused a significant increase in carbonylated fibrinogen at the end of dialysis compared to the start of dialysis, whereas there was no change with the 62.5 mg dose or during dialysis without iron treatment. The authors concluded that 125 mg dose of ferric gluconate should be used with caution [80]. In a study of 71 hemodialysis and peritoneal dialysis patients treated routinely with intravenous iron preparations, 20% of the patients had detectable labile plasma iron that was found to be persistently elevated in 12 of the patients for at least 2 months. The authors concluded that some patients may be exposed to a persistent, low level of labile plasma iron [29]. Recently, the relationship between the use of intravenous iron sucrose, advanced oxidation protein products (AOPP – a marker of oxidant-mediated protein damage), and CA-IMT was explored in 79 stage 5 CKD hemodialysis patients. The cumulative iron dose was positively related to CA-IMT in patients < 60 years old and with AOPP in the entire study population [26]. In the aggregate, these studies suggest that all intravenous iron preparations likely have the potential to induce oxidative stress, and that free iron may lead to atherosclerosis.

How oxidative stress is related to plaque instability in stage 5 CKD is not quite clear, but several mechanisms potentially play a role. Oxidation of the LDL moiety appears to be a major event leading to the uptake of LDL by the macrophage, and represents but one potential effect of increased oxidative stress in these patients. In addition, superoxide might increase the expression of metalloproteinases (MMP) in the foam cells and thus promoting plaque instability. It has been suggested that MMPs contribute to vascular remodeling during the development and progression of human atherosclerosis; more specifically MMP2 and MMP9 are noted to be increased in human coronary arteries, as well as in abdominal aortic aneurysms [37]. MMPs produced by macrophage-derived foam cells include MMP-1, MMP-2, MMP-3, as well as MMP-7. Axisa et al. [8] have shown doxycycline, a MMP inhibitor, penetrates atherosclerotic plaques and results in a reduction in MMP-1 concentration, because of decreased expression. Such inhibitors of MMPs may promote plaque stability, and may provide a possible therapeutic venue in the future. MMPs may be increased in patients with stage 5 CKD as compared to the general population. Ebihara et al. [27] reported an enhanced expression of MMP-9 mRNA in 60 stage 5 CKD patients as compared to healthy controls. Of note, this increase was not demonstrated in the 20 patients with CKD not yet requiring dialysis who were included in the study. The enhanced MMP-9 expression did not seem to be related to the dialysis procedure itself, although it was noted to be more pronounced in patients on hemodialysis rather than on peritoneal dialysis. Thus, it is possible that MMPs act as modulators of the atherosclerotic process in patients with stage 5 CKD, and that their expression may be enhanced by oxidative stress (Figure 1).

Myeloperoxidase is one of the most abundant enzymes in the phagocyte, it is rapidly secreted upon stimulation, and catalyzes halides to their corresponding hypohalous. Catalytically active myeloperoxidase has been identified in atherosclerotic tissue, and found to co-localize with foamy cells [46]. It is also linked to modulation of vascular signaling and the vasodilatory functions of NO, impairing endothelium-dependant relaxation [126]. A recent study has shown that an elevated leukocyte count and myeloperoxidase level are associated increased CA-IMT in a large group of non-CKD patients [131.143]. A case control study including 158 patients with established CAD and 175 patients without angiographically significant CAD found that leukocyte- and blood-MPO levels were both significantly greater in patients with CAD than in controls. In multivariable models adjusting for traditional cardiovascular risk factors, Framingham risk score, and white blood cell counts, MPO levels were significantly associated with presence of CAD [143]. Limited information is available concerning the correlation between MPO levels and cardiovascular disease in kidney disease patients. In a study of a cohort of 155 stage 5 CKD patients shortly prior to the initiation of dialysis treatment, a functional variant of the MPO gene GG was found to be associated with cardiovascular disease in stage 5 CKD patients [93]. Not surprisingly, these patients had higher plasma levels of the AGE pentosidine than controls. Myeloperoxidase has been linked to the production of AGEs thru increased production of aldehydes [46].

Carbonyl Stress

A variety of oxidative reactions, including the addition of oxygen to the unsaturated carbon double bonds in carbohydrates, lipids or amino acids, can lead to the formation of aldehydes as the end-product. Detection of aldehydes relies on identification of the carbonyl group of the molecule, leading to the term "carbonyl stress." These reactive carbonyl compounds are important in the generation of AGEs and ALEs. Advanced glycation is initiated by nonenzymatic reactions between reactive carbonyl compounds and various amino groups in proteins. Rearrangement reactions take place to produce AGEs that remain irreversibly bound to proteins, are highly reactive, and appear to be cleared at least in part, by the kidney [17]. Decreased clearance in patients with kidney disease has been implicated as one of the reasons AGEs are elevated in patients with CKD. On the other hand, increased de novo synthesis due to oxidative stress and accumulations of reactive precursors, such as di-carbonyls, has been implicated as well [46,69]. AGEs may promote atherosclerosis through interactions with specific receptors (RAGE), causing increased expression of adhesion molecules and enhanced attraction of circulating monocytes. They also seem to increase the production of IL-6 and CRP, and hence may provide a link between oxidative stress and inflammation in atherosclerosis [46]. There is also evidence that AGEs may modify LDL making it less amenable to clearance by the LDL receptors [17]. Bucala et al. [17] demonstrated that AGE-modified LDL exhibited markedly impaired clearance kinetics when injected into transgenic mice expressing the human LDL receptor.

The importance of AGEs in the pathogenesis of atherosclerosis in stage 5 CKD patients has evolved from several observations. First, levels of AGEs from the arteries of dialysis patients are higher than in normal subjects [76]. Second, high levels of immunoreactive AGE accumulates at high levels in diabetic and aged vascular intima, particularly along the inner elastic layer of arteries [89]. Another immunohistochemical study demonstrated increased AGE accumulation in the aortic wall of diabetic and non-diabetic stage 5 CKD patients as compared to controls [100], highlighting the potential role these products may play in the atherosclerotic process, regardless of the presence or absence of diabetes. Interestingly, a cross sectional study by Schwedler et al. [106] not only failed to reveal a predictive role for serum AGEs on mortality in stage 5 CKD patients, but also found that high serum AGEs partly overcame the negative impact of the acute phase response on mortality in hemodialysis patients. Based on these data, high serum AGEs levels in stage 5 CKD patients may be simply an epiphenomenon accompanying underlying atherosclerosis, or the higher levels may reflect better nutritional support of these patients. Additional studies are needed to assess the potential role AGEs may play in the cardiovascular mortality in these patients [107], and to define more clearly the relationship between inflammation and oxidative stress in stage 5 CKD patients. Whether increased oxidative stress is a direct mediator of the accelerated atherosclerotic process in stage 5 CKD patients with markedly elevated acute phase reactants, or whether it is --- as argued by some --- merely an epiphenomenon accompanying the establishment of atherosclerosis remains unclear.

Impaired Nitric Oxide Bioavailability

Nitric oxide (NO) is a potent vasodilator, cell signaling molecule, and proinflammatory agent critical for many functions in the vasculature and kidney [62-64] that also inhibits key processes of atherosclerosis, including monocyte-endothelial adhesion, platelet aggregation, and vascular smooth muscle cell proliferation. Hence, endothelial dysfunction related to reduced bioavailability of NO is an early step in the course of atherosclerosis. NO is synthesized from the amino acid L-arginine by the action of NO synthases (NOS). NOS isoenzymes can be blocked by endogenous competitive inhibitors, such as asymmetric dimethylarginine (ADMA) [34]. Endothelial cells can elaborate ADMA, which can impair endothelium-dependent vasodilation and leukocyte adhesion. ADMA is metabolized by dimethylarginine dimethylaminohydrolase (DDAH) into citrulline and dimethylamine (Figure2).

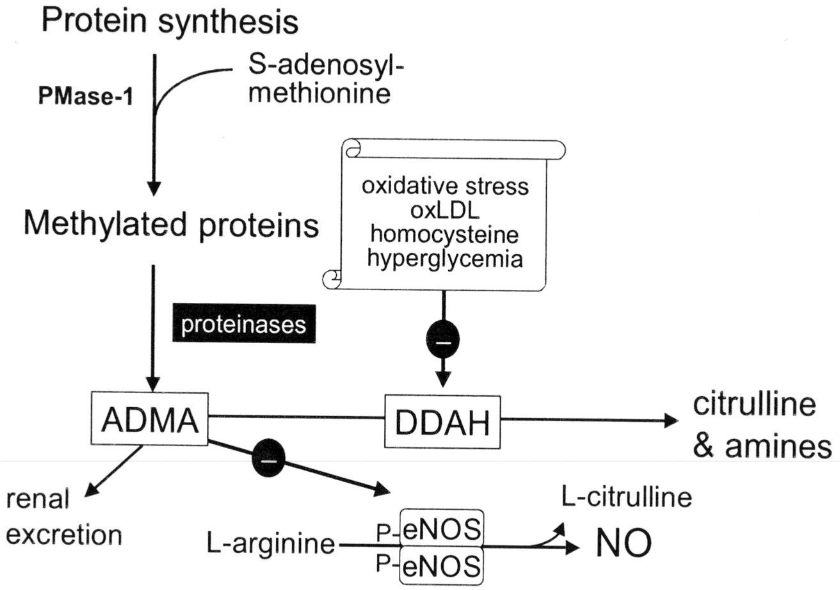

Figure 2. Pathways for formation, degradation, and clearance of asymmetric dimethylarginine (ADMA). ADMA, a competitive inhibitor of nitric oxide synthases (NOS), is synthesized by protein-arginine methyltransferases (PMase), a family of enzymes that methylate L-arginine residues within target proteins. ADMA is metabolized by dimethylarginine dimethylaminohydrolase (DDAH), and inhibition of DDAH activity leads to increased ADMA levels, inhibition of endothelial NOS (eNOS), and endothelial dysfunction. Blood levels of ADMA are increased in advanced chronic kidney disease, atherosclerosis, hypercholesterolemia, and hyperhomocysteinemia.

Patients with CKD have reduced NO bioavailability [94]. This reduction in NO levels correlates with increased serum ADMA levels in stage 5 CKD patients as compared to the general population [59,103,136]. Interestingly, Kielestein et al. [60] demonstrated ADMA levels to be equally increased in 44 nonsmoking nondiabetic patients with confirmed primary kidney disease, regardless of whether their CKD was mild, moderate or advanced. Similar results were documented by Fleck et al. [33], who studied 221 patients with CKD at different stages. Conceptually, this increase in ADMA levels early in the course of CKD is likely to contribute to the increased cardiovascular mortality secondary to atherosclerosis in this group of patients. The reason behind this increase in ADMA is not clear. Since ADMA is only partially cleared by the kidney, and because its levels start to rise even in the face of only mild CKD, reduced clearance cannot solely account for the marked elevations of its level in such patients. Theoretically, as the kidney disease progresses, and with continued loss of renal tissue (containing DDAH), impairment of ADMA degradation by this organ can occur, leading to its increased availability [34]. Regardless of the mechanism(s) responsible for the higher concentrations of ADMA in this patient population, ADMA, at the reported concentrations is capable of inhibiting NO production.

ADMA has recently emerged as an important risk factor for cardiovascular disease and mortality in stage 5 CKD. Zocalli et al. [146] investigated increased ADMA levels as a risk factor for cardiovascular disease in CKD patients in a prospective study involving a cohort of 225 hemodialysis patients, and found that ADMA was a strong and independent predictor of overall mortality and cardiovascular outcome in stage 5 CKD. Furthermore, in a separate study of 90 patients on hemodialysis, his group found that higher levels of ADMA were associated with higher CA-IMT at baseline, as well as with greater progression of the atherosclerotic lesion [145]. In that study, multiple regression analysis indicated that the interaction between ADMA and CRP was the sole independent predictor of the progression of intimal lesions, suggesting a link between ADMA and inflammation. Oxidative stress has been shown to increase the activity of arginine methylating and ADMA-degrading enzymes leading to increased ADMA concentrations [6,130]. The exact mechanism by which this occurs is unclear, and further research is needed to define the relationship between inflammation, oxidative stress and ADMA.

Decreased NO bioavailability in patients with CKD may potentially be mediated by other factors than those altering ADMA levels. For example, Moeslinger and Spieckermann [82] analyzed the effect of urea on iNOS and macrophage proliferation. According to their results, urea caused a dose-dependant reduction in iNOS protein levels and NO produced by RAW 264.7 macrophage cells. This was accompanied by increased cell proliferation. Furthermore Jankowski et al. [52] found that phenyl acetic acid, which is present at higher levels in the blood of stage 5 CKD patients, inhibits iNOS expression in mononuclear leukocytes. These studies suggest that urea and other uremic toxins may exert an inhibitory effect on NO production in vivo.

Malnutrition

Protein energy malnutrition (PEM), a state of decreased pool of body proteins with or without fat depletion, is estimated to affect 50% of stage 5 CKD dialysis patients. The speculated causes of PEM in this patient population are several [55]. Hypoalbuminemia, hypotransferrinemia and hypocholesterolemia are considered clinical indicators of PEM. Hypoalbuminemia, in particular, has been associated with increased cardiovascular mortality in dialysis patients; several studies have shown that for each 1 g/dl decrement in albumin, the cardiovascular mortality increases by 31%. Cardiovascular mortality in these studies included atherosclerotic as well as non-atherosclerotic complications. Furthermore, few studies have attempted to evaluate a temporal relationship between lower albumin levels and cardiovascular complications [55]. Ng et al. [10] reviewed data abstracted from 5,058 patients with stage 5 CKD who participated in the USRDS Dialysis Morbidity and Mortality Study Wave. As indicated in prior studies, with the decrement of albumin, the cardiovascular mortality increased even in the patients who had no evidence of cardiovascular complications at baseline [36].

Albumin is believed to provide strong antioxidant protection, and may function as a suicide scavenger preventing oxidative injury to lipoproteins and the vessel wall. According to some authors, a low plasma albumin signifies a markedly diminished antioxidant capacity, thus participating in the process of atherosclerosis in this patient population [46]. Moreover, Himmelfarb et al. [45] demonstrated that albumin is the main target for carbonyl formation in uremic patients. Analysis of 9,250 U.S. adults aged 30-74 years who participated in the Second National Health and Nutrition Examination Survey (NHANES II) revealed that elevated WBC count and hypoalbuminemia were associated with future risk for CKD, supporting the hypothesis that systemic inflammation is an independent risk factor for CKD [28].

PEM may contribute to the atherosclerotic process in CKD patients via other mechanisms. For example, stage 5 CKD patients have inadequate intake of L-arginine, a substrate for NO, thus leading to lower NO levels. In addition, albumin is normally a protein reservoir for NO, so that as albumin levels decline, the metabolism of NO may be hastened [36]. Poor nutrition also is associated with an increase in Lp(a), another risk factors for atherosclerosis. In any event, the exact relationship between PEM, inflammation and atherosclerosis remains incompletely defined and deserves further scrutiny.

Hyperhomocysteinemia

Homocysteine is a metabolic product of methyl group donation by the amino acid methionine. Moderate elevation of plasma homocysteine (> 15 μM) is most commonly caused by deficiencies of B-vitamins, such as folic acid, B6 and B12. Genetic factors, drugs, and renal impairment also play a role. Homocysteine has several deleterious vascular actions. It increases oxidant stress, impairs NO synthesis, and is toxic to endothelial cells, promoting their adhesion with neutrophils. Homocysteine also may promote thrombosis by indirectly activating endothelial cell factor V and inactivating protein C and thrombomodulin. A significant body of epidemiological evidence suggests that hyperhomocysteinemia acts as an independent risk factor for atherosclerosis in the general population [43].

Moderate hyperhomocysteinemia is present in >90% of stage 5 CKD patients [84]. The underlying cause of this high prevalence is unclear, since renal excretion of homocysteine accounts for only 1% of its clearance. Nutritional deficiencies in such patients are common; however, it is also noted in these patients that vitamin supplementation does not normalize the homocysteine levels. Inflammation and the high incidence of diabetes in this group of patients may also play a role. Despite the common occurrence of hyperhomocysteinemia in these patients, the correlation between elevated homocysteine levels and cardiovascular mortality in CKD patients is controversial [128]. Moustapha et al. [85] reported a graded association between the risk for cardiovascular events and plasma total homocysteine levels in stage 5 CKD patients over 17 months of follow up. In a prospective study by Bostom et al. [16], plasma total homocysteine levels greater than or equal to 27 μM compared to levels less than 27 μM were associated with a relative risk of 3-4 for cardiovascular events in patients with stage 5 CKD. Other small studies have also demonstrated an association between atherosclerosis and hyperhomocysteinemia [129,142]. On the other hand, Suliman et al. [128] reported that CKD patients with cardiovascular disease to have lower plasma total homocysteine levels. However, it is possible that this paradoxical relationship in this report relates to the high prevalence of hypoalbuminemia in the patients with the lower plasma total homocysteine levels. While it is likely that hyperhomocysteinemia does contribute to the atherosclerotic process in stage 5 CKD patients, the multiple coexisting risk factors in such patients, make it difficult to prove this hypothesis in the clinical studies.

Chronic Anemia

Anemia is a common, and frequently under-treated, condition among CKD patients, especially in the pre-dialysis stages of CKD. Anemia is associated with a markedly increased risk of death in the stage 5 CKD patient population, and is recognized as an independent predictor of cardiovascular events in this group of patients [3]. Data on 13,716 participants followed for 9 years in the prospective Atherosclerosis Risk In Communities (ARIC) study suggest that the presence of both CKD (stages 1 to 4) and anemia is associated with a substantial increase in stroke risk, independent of other risk factors for stroke [3]. Further analysis of 15,792 patients derived from the same study population (ARIC) and followed for 9 years indicated that patients with no baseline cardiac disease but with anemia (defined as hemoglobin of <13mg/dl for men and <12mg/dl for women), a higher serum creatinine was predictive of higher risk of ischemic cardiac disease [54]. It is possible, however, that the anemia may only be a reflection of the duration and severity of the underlying CKD, or that both cardiovascular disease and anemia result from the underlying inflammation and oxidative stress secondary to the CKD. This possibility is especially important since there are relationships between anemia, inflammation, and oxidative stress. For example, after an inflammatory response to an infection, hemoglobin levels decrease within 2-3 days, mainly because of a reduction in erythrocyte survival [119]. In addition to that, serum from uremic patients has been noted to inhibit erythroid colony formation in response to erythropoietin, a process that can be reversed by the addition of antibodies to tumor necrosis factor-α (TNF-α) and interferon-γ (IFN-γ) [5]. However, it should also be noted that anemia is potentially associated with increased oxidative stress, as observed from the increased plasma concentrations of some of the markers of oxidative stress, such as malonyldialdehyde, in CKD patients [75].

The available evidence indicates that anemia is more likely the result of the underlying inflammation associated with CKD, and it may result in increased oxidative stress, and thereby contribute to endothelial cell dysfunction and the atherosclerotic process. The exact relationship between IV iron therapy, erythropoietin replacement and mortality deserves further investigative scrutiny.

Vascular Calcification

In the past, it was considered that vascular calcification was a passive degenerative process, but recent data have shown that vessel wall calcification is an active and regulated process, sharing some similarities with osteogenesis [81,111]. Endochondral bone formation has been demonstrated in the hearts of oopherectomized aged female rats, suggesting that vascular calcification may be yet another mechanism associated with the development of atherosclerosis [32]. The presence of arterial wall calcification has been demonstrated in association with atherosclerosis in the general population, especially with increased age [126,134]. Coronary artery calcification, detected by EBCT, has been demonstrated in stage 5 CKD dialysis patients who are even younger than 30 years of age [40]. Merjanian et al. [78] showed in a group of diabetic patients with CKD that coronary artery as well as valvular calcification was evident and often advanced even before progression to stage 5 CKD requiring dialysis. With the EBCT scanner, vascular calcification scores in dialysis patients can double in 14 months. Two types of vascular calcification have been described: intimal and medial. Arterial intimal calcification represents an advanced stage of atherosclerosis, seems to be associated with plaque development in patients with the traditional risk factors for atherosclerosis, and it is present in patients stage 5 CKD. Acute medial calcification is associated with aging, the presence and the duration of diabetes, and it is commonly present in patients with stage 5 CKD [71].

Vascular calcification has been associated with increased cardiovascular risk and all-cause mortality in both the general population and in patients with CKD [126,137]. London et al. [71] demonstrated that both arterial intimal calcification and arterial medial calcification are strong, independent prognostic markers for all cause mortality in stage 5 CKD patients. Their results also suggested that factors other than the duration of dialysis, including calcium and phosphorus metabolism, and possibly inflammation and malnutrition, were responsible for this phenomenon, since patients with lower serum albumin and higher CRP were more likely to have either type of calcification. Other studies have found hyperphosphatemia, calcium X phosphorus product and hyperparathyroidism to be independently associated with an increased risk of death from cardiovascular disease in stage 5 CKD patients [13,58]. Daily phosphate and calcium balances become positive in the late stages of CKD, when the GFR declines below 30-25 ml/min. Use of dietary phosphate binders that are calcium-based likely further contributes to positive calcium balances. The non-calcium-based phosphate binder sevelamer hydrochloride is as efficacious as calcium-based phosphate binders for reducing serum phosphorus but does not promote hypercalcemia. Sevelamer also consistently and significantly decreases LDL cholesterol and increases HDL cholesterol in most studies. In a randomized clinical trial comparing sevelamer and calcium-based binders, both agents yielded excellent phosphorus control, but calcium-based binders led to significantly higher serum calcium concentrations and to the progression of coronary artery and aortic calcification, whereas sevelamer did not produce hypercalcemia and attenuated or arrested progression of vascular progression [20]. Interestingly, even in non-CKD patients, there seems to be a correlation between serum phosphate levels and vascular calcification, underscoring the importance of phosphate in this process [31].

The relationship between vascular calcification and atherosclerosis has been further explored by Wang et al. [138], who studied 137 patients on continuous ambulatory peritoneal dialysis (CAPD) and found that patients with vascular calcification had higher levels of CRP, and lower levels of albumin. Another cross-sectional study in 312 hemodialysis patients found that higher CRP levels were associated with lower levels of α2-Heremans-Schmid glycoprotein/fetuin (AHSg/fetuin), an important circulating inhibitor of calcification in vivo. AHSg/fetuin is also considered a negative acute phase reactant [65]. Another interesting phenomenon is that AHSg/fetuin knockout mice develop excessive vascular calcification of a metastatic pattern, involving the parenchyma of several organs; such as lung and the heart [58]. In the aggregate, these data suggest that vascular calcification in patients with CKD may be enhanced further by their persistent state of chronic inflammation (Figure 1). Matrix G1α protein (MGP) is another calcium-regulating protein that has sparked recent interest. It is noted that MGP knockout mice develop arterial medial calcification in the abdominal aorta, presumable secondary to the unopposed osteogenic activity on the vascular mesenchyme [25]. What role this may play in patients with CKD is unclear.

Therapeutic Options

Traditional Risk Factors

Considering the fact that atherosclerosis is the principal cause of excess mortality in patients with CKD, it is important to manage aggressively cardiovascular risk factors in these patients. In addition, the pathogenesis of atherosclerosis and CKD share several common antecedents. Identifying the multiple risk factors that account for the development of atherosclerosis provides several targets for current and future therapies. It is sobering that in such patients, epidemiological evidence suggests that even the traditional risk factors are inadequately managed. In addition, it is important to recognize that the life span of most CKD patients exceeds the duration of treatment required for the beneficial effect of risk factor reduction on morbidity and mortality.

In patients with the earlier stages of CKD (stages 1 through 4), several studies have indicated that appropriate management of hypertension not only slows the progression of CKD, but also reduces the risk of ischemic cardiac events and related mortality. The NKF task force recommends that patients with CKD should be considered in the highest-risk group for cardiovascular disease events, irrespective of traditional cardiovascular disease risk factors. Similarly, JNC-7 recommends lower target blood pressure and angiotensin converting enzyme inhibitors or angiotensin II receptor blockers for CKD patients, primarily due to their beneficial effect of delaying progression of CKD in addition to reducing hypertension. According to the 7th report of the JNC, target blood pressure to achieve this goal in patients with CKD and proteinuria >1g/d should be <125/75 [21]. It is currently incompletely understood what role hypertension plays in increasing the risk of cardiovascular death in individuals with stage 5 CKD, or what blood pressure levels should be targeted in the management of this patient group. It seems appropriate to tailor the management of hypertension individually in such patients, taking into account other co-morbidities, such as stroke or cardiomyopathy, in addition to the number of episodes of intra and inter-dialytic hypotension and the patient's quality of life [135]. The choice of antihypertensive agent should also take into account these factors although one might argue that ACEIs or ARBs should be the first line of therapy, because of their possible favorable effect on endothelial dysfunction.

The benefit of lipid-lowering therapy on cardiovascular outcome has not been proven in randomized controlled intervention trials in CKD patients. Current practice recommendations are extrapolated from clinical studies in the general population, but it remains possible that such results may not be applicable to all patients with CKD. Moreover, it is possible that treatment of dyslipidemias may not be as safe or effective in some subpopulations of CKD patients. Nonetheless, according to the recently published "NKF-K/DOQI Clinical Practice Guidelines on Managing Dyslipidemia in Chronic Kidney Disease," all patients with CKD should be included in the highest-risk group and have lower target LDL levels.

There is increasing evidence that the cardio-protective effects of statins in the general population are derived not only from their lipid-lowering effect [67], but also their anti-inflammatory effects that may promote plaque stability [127]. In human monocytes in vitro, statins have been shown to inhibit the DNA binding activity of NF-κB, an important transcription factor involved in the activation of early genes during inflammation [44]. There is also evidence that they reduce leukocyte adhesion and macrophage activation and alter human plaque content leading to less expression of MMPs, thereby increasing plaque stability [24]. Further, they have been shown to have potent antioxidant effects by limiting production of myeloperoxidase- and NO-derived oxidants [112]. The effects of statins on cardiovascular mortality in stage 5 CKD patients has only been examined in observational studies; in these analyses, these agents have been shown to be associated with lower mortality in patients with stage 5 CKD [110]. Short-term randomized controlled trials have shown that statins are safe and effective in lowering total cholesterol and LDL cholesterol levels in patients with stage 5 CKD [42, 49, 101]. Additional randomized, placebo-controlled trials on lipid-lowering therapy and cardiovascular outcome in CKD patients are clearly needed. One currently ongoing study, the AURORA study, is designed to examine the effects of rosuvastatin in approximately 3000 male and female dialysis patients with the objective of demonstrating an effect on cardiovascular mortality and morbidity [30].

Inflammation, Oxidative Stress and Endothelial Dysfunction as Potential Therapeutic Targets

Unlike dyslipidemias, there are no intervention trials from patients in the general (or CKD) population that conclusively demonstrate that modification of non-traditional risk factors reduces cardiovascular disease. Moreover, it remains possible that results of clinical trials conduced in the general population may not be applicable to all patients with CKD. The recent understanding of the roles played by inflammation, oxidative stress and endothelial dysfunction in the pathogenesis of atherosclerosis opens new doors for possible therapeutic options in preventing or slowing the accelerated process of atherosclerosis in CKD patients. Several agents, namely ACE inhibitors, PPAR agonists and antioxidants may be of benefit in targeting these nontraditional risk factors.

Angiotensin II Inhibition

Mounting evidence indicates that angiotensin II is involved in promoting vascular inflammation. In the apoE-deficient mice, treatment with angiotensin II leads to NF-κB activation, accelerated atherosclerosis, and aneurysm formation [133]. Angiotensin II is also thought to promote endothelial and smooth muscle cell expression of IL-6, and to increase plaque instability by stimulating growth factors, cytokines, and MMPs [104]. Thus, it is not surprising that reducing angiotensin II production with ACEIs, or blocking its actions with ARBs, would help improve endothelial function and retard atherogenesis both in the general population and in patients with CKD. Furthermore, ACEIs seem to enhance endothelial elaboration of and the bioactivity of NO, which would also contribute to the beneficial effects of these drugs [108]. While these drugs have been shown to reduce inflammatory markers in patients with pre-dialysis CKD [122], their potential benefit in slowing the progression of atherosclerosis patients with stage 5 CKD remains to be tested in a proper randomized controlled trial.

Peroxisome Proliferator-Activated Receptor (PPAR) Agonists

PPARs are transcription factors that regulate expression of numerous genes affecting glycemic control, lipid metabolism, vascular tone and inflammation. Downregulation of PPAR by pro-inflammatory molecules, such as angiotensin II, may aggravate further vascular inflammation and atherosclerosis. In vitro studies suggest that PPAR stimulation may have anti-inflammatory effects and may suppress the generation of ROS [83]. A recent clinical study examining the effect of the PPAR agonist rosiglitazone on traditional and nontraditional risk factors of cardiovascular disease in type II diabetics demonstrated a reduction in the levels of MMP-9 and CRP, suggesting that this drug may play a role in modulating the inflammatory response associated with the atherosclerotic process in these individuals. Whether these medications can be utilized safely and effectively in patients with CKD will require further investigation.

Antioxidants

Despite the fact that several studies have failed to demonstrate an improvement in cardiovascular outcome in non-renal patients taking vitamin E [1,73], vitamin E may still play a role in modulating the atherosclerotic process in CKD patients. It is likely that CKD patients, especially in the advanced stages, are under a significant amount of oxidative stress, potentially rendering them more likely to benefit from this agent than other patient groups. The Secondary Prevention with Antioxidants of Cardiovascular Disease in End-Stage Renal Disease (SPACE) Study randomized 196 stage 5 CKD hemodialysis patients with pre-existing coronary artery disease to receive either 800 U of vitamin E or placebo daily. The vitamin E group had a lower incidence of the primary end point, which was a composite of fatal or nonfatal myocardial infarction, ischemic stroke, peripheral vascular disease, and unstable angina [14]. Recently, vitamin E-bonded hemodialyzers have been developed, and they have been shown to reduce levels of IL-6, and improve endothelial function during hemodialysis. There is also evidence that they may be beneficial at reducing atherosclerosis, as indexed by their favorable effects on CA-IMT [61].

In another recent controlled trial, 134 stage 5 CKD hemodialysis patients were randomized to either 600 mg of oral acetylcysteine (an antioxidant) twice per day or placebo [132]. Those patients randomized to acetylcysteine experienced a lower incidence of the primary end point, which was a composite of myocardial infarction, death attributable to cardiovascular disease, need for coronary intervention, ischemic stroke, and peripheral vascular disease. Although these clinical studies should be interpreted with caution because a small population was studied and the results were contrary to studies in the general population, given the fact that stage 5 CKD patients have greater oxidant stress and inflammation than the general population, the results should be followed up in larger trials. Clearly, other antioxidants would need to be evaluated in this group of patients, as they may confer greater benefit. It is also important to note that vitamin C intake higher than 500 mg per day in the setting of CKD should be avoided, because vitamin C can crystallize with oxalate in the renal parenchyma to aggravate renal injury.

Homocysteine

All CKD patients should be screened for hyperhomocysteinemia. If total homocysteine levels are elevated, CKD patients should be counseled to commence high dose folic acid therapy. Although low doses of folic acid (0.4 mg per day) are effective in lowering plasma homocysteine levels in the general population, much higher doses are required for therapeutic effect in most CKD patients. The most effective reduction in total plasma homocysteine levels in CKD patients comes from a combination of high dose daily folic acid (15 mg), B6 (100 mg), and B12 (100 mcg).

Vascular Calcification

Since vascular calcification is linked to increased cardiovascular mortality and advanced atherosclerosis in CKD, controlling the rate of calcification would appear pertinent to slow down this process in our patients. As of today, there is no effective therapy for reversing vascular calcification; hence there is much focus on preventing it through the aggressive control of hyperphosphatemia, calcium X phosphorus product and parathyroid hormone levels in these patients. The K/DOQI guidelines dictate target phosphorus levels of <5.5mg/dl, calcium X phosphorus product <55, and the PTH level in the range of 150-300 pg/ml for stage 5 CKD patients, utilizing phosphate binders and vitamin D analogs, and expert dietary counsel to maintain dietary phosphate intake less than 1-1.2 grams per day in order to achieve these goal levels.

Conclusions

Given the high incidence of ischemic cardiovascular disease and related mortality in patients with CKD, considerable research effort should be made at the bench and in the clinics to distinguish distinctive pathogenetic mechanisms responsible for the accelerated atherosclerosis in these individuals and effective preventive treatments. With the recognition that cardiovascular mortality is increased even in the earlier stages of CKD, traditional and non-traditional risk factors need to be addressed more aggressively, both in terms of their role in advancing atherosclerosis and as potential management targets. Further research is required in CKD patients to characterize vascular morphology in the different vascular beds, establish the pathogenetic mechanisms of vascular and plaque calcification, test the potential beneficial effect of rigorous control of non-traditional risk factors, and the superimposed role of diabetes mellitus in amplifying these vascular alterations. Although no definitive good therapy has been identified to aid in treating such patients, the use of certain agents such ACE inhibitors, ARBs, and statins does seem to improve their poor outcome, and should be advocated. Clearly, further studies are needed to help guide our management of atherosclerotic cardiovascular disease in CKD patients.

References

[1] The HOPE (Heart Outcomes Prevention Evaluation) Study: the design of a large, simple randomized trial of an angiotensin-converting enzyme inhibitor (ramipril) and vitamin E in patients at high risk of cardiovascular events. The HOPE study investigators. *Can J Cardiol 12*: 127-137, 1996.

[2] National Kidney Foundation K/DOQI clinical practice guidelines on managing dyslipidemias in chronic kidney disease. *Am J Kidney Dis 41 (suppl 3):* S1-S77, 2003.

[3] Abramson JL, Jurkovitz CT, Vaccarino V, Weintraub WS, and McClellan W. Chronic kidney disease, anemia, and incident stroke in a middle-aged, community-based population: the ARIC Study. *Kidney Int 64*: 610-615, 2003.

[4] Agewall S and Bjorn F. Microalbuminuria and intima-media thickness of the carotid artery in clinically healthy men. *Atherosclerosis 164*: 161-166, 2002.

[5] Allen DA, Breen C, Yaqoob MM, and Macdougall IC. Inhibition of CFU-E colony formation in uremic patients with inflammatory disease: role of IFN-gamma and TNF-alpha. *J Investig Med 47*: 204-211, 1999.

[6] Annuk M, Zilmer M, and Fellstrom B. Endothelium-dependent vasodilation and oxidative stress in chronic renal failure: impact on cardiovascular disease. *Kidney Int Suppl:* S50-53, 2003.

[7] Ashman N, Macey MG, Fan SL, Azam U, and Yaqoob MM. Increased platelet-monocyte aggregates and cardiovascular disease in end-stage renal failure patients. *Nephrol Dial Transplant 18*: 2088-2096, 2003.

[8] Axisa B, Loftus IM, Naylor AR, Goodall S, Jones L, Bell PR, and Thompson MM. Prospective, randomized, double-blind trial investigating the effect of doxycycline on matrix metalloproteinase expression within atherosclerotic carotid plaques. *Stroke 33*: 2858-2864, 2002.

[9] Balla J, Vercellotti GM, Nath K, Yachie A, Nagy E, Eaton JW, and Balla G. Haem, haem oxygenase and ferritin in vascular endothelial cell injury. *Nephrol Dial Transplant 18 Suppl 5*: v8-12, 2003.

[10] Beddhu S, Kaysen GA, Yan G, Sarnak M, Agodoa L, Ornt D, and Cheung AK. Association of serum albumin and atherosclerosis in chronic hemodialysis patients. *Am J Kidney Dis 40:* 721-727, 2002.

[11] Blankenberg S, Luc G, Ducimetiere P, Arveiler D, Ferrieres J, Amouyel P, Evans A, Cambien F, and Tiret L. Interleukin-18 and the risk of coronary heart disease in European men: the Prospective Epidemiological Study of Myocardial Infarction (PRIME). *Circulation 108*: 2453-2459, 2003.

[12] Blankenberg S, Tiret L, Bickel C, Peetz D, Cambien F, Meyer J, and Rupprecht HJ. Interleukin-18 is a strong predictor of cardiovascular death in stable and unstable angina. *Circulation 106*: 24-30, 2002.

[13] Block GA, Hulbert-Shearon TE, Levin NW, and Port FK. Association of serum phosphorus and calcium x phosphate product with mortality risk in chronic hemodialysis patients: a national study. *Am J Kidney Dis 31*: 607-617, 1998.

[14] Boaz M, Smetana S, Weinstein T, Matas Z, Gafter U, Iaina A, Knecht A, Weissgarten Y, Brunner D, Fainaru M, and Green MS. Secondary prevention with antioxidants of cardiovascular disease in endstage renal disease (SPACE): randomised placebo-controlled trial. *Lancet 356*: 1213-1218, 2000.

[15] Bostom AG, Gagnon DR, Cupples LA, Wilson PW, Jenner JL, Ordovas JM, Schaefer EJ, and Castelli WP. A prospective investigation of elevated lipoprotein (a) detected by electrophoresis and cardiovascular disease in women. The Framingham Heart Study. *Circulation 90:* 1688-1695, 1994.

[16] Bostom AG, Shemin D, Verhoef P, Nadeau MR, Jacques PF, Selhub J, Dworkin L, and Rosenberg IH. Elevated fasting total plasma homocysteine levels and cardiovascular disease outcomes in maintenance dialysis patients. A prospective study. *Arterioscler Thromb Vasc Biol 17*: 2554-2558, 1997.

[17] Bucala R, Makita Z, Vega G, Grundy S, Koschinsky T, Cerami A, and Vlassara H. Modification of low density lipoprotein by advanced glycation end products contributes to the dyslipidemia of diabetes and renal insufficiency. *Proc Natl Acad Sci U S A 91*: 9441-9445, 1994.

[18] Cai H and Harrison DG. Endothelial dysfunction in cardiovascular diseases: the role of oxidant stress. *Circ Res 87*: 840-844, 2000.

[19] Caligiuri G, Rudling M, Ollivier V, Jacob MP, Michel JB, Hansson GK, and Nicoletti A. Interleukin-10 deficiency increases atherosclerosis, thrombosis, and low-density lipoproteins in apolipoprotein E knockout mice. *Mol Med 9*: 10-17, 2003.

[20] Chertow GM, Raggi P, McCarthy JT, Schulman G, Silberzweig J, Kuhlik A, Goodman WG, Boulay A, Burke SK, and Toto RD. The effects of sevelamer and calcium acetate on proxies of atherosclerotic and arteriosclerotic vascular disease in hemodialysis patients. *Am J Nephrol 23*: 307-314, 2003.

[21] Chobanian AV, Bakris GL, Black HR, Cushman WC, Green LA, Izzo JL, Jr., Jones DW, Materson BJ, Oparil S, Wright JT, Jr., and Roccella EJ. Seventh report of the Joint National Committee on Prevention, Detection, Evaluation, and Treatment of High Blood Pressure. *Hypertension 42*: 1206-1252, 2003.

[22] Coresh J, Wei GL, McQuillan G, Brancati FL, Levey AS, Jones C, and Klag MJ. Prevalence of high blood pressure and elevated serum creatinine level in the United States: findings from the third National Health and Nutrition Examination Survey (1988-1994). *Arch Intern Med 161*: 1207-1216, 2001.

[23] Cressman MD, Heyka RJ, Paganini EP, O'Neil J, Skibinski CI, and Hoff HF. Lipoprotein(a) is an independent risk factor for cardiovascular disease in hemodialysis patients. *Circulation 86*: 475-482, 1992.

[24] Crisby M, Nordin-Fredriksson G, Shah PK, Yano J, Zhu J, and Nilsson J. Pravastatin treatment increases collagen content and decreases lipid content, inflammation, metalloproteinases, and cell death in human carotid plaques: implications for plaque stabilization. *Circulation 103*: 926-933, 2001.

[25] Demer LL, Tintut Y, and Parhami F. Novel mechanisms in accelerated vascular calcification in renal disease patients. *Curr Opin Nephrol Hypertens 11*: 437-443, 2002.

[26] Drueke T, Witko-Sarsat V, Massy Z, Descamps-Latscha B, Guerin AP, Marchais SJ, Gausson V, and London GM. Iron therapy, advanced oxidation protein products, and carotid artery intima-media thickness in end-stage renal disease. *Circulation 106*: 2212-2217, 2002.

[27] Ebihara I, Nakamura T, Tomino Y, Shimada N, and Koide H. Metalloproteinase-9 mRNA expression in monocytes from patients with chronic renal failure. *Am J Nephrol 18*: 305-310, 1998.

[28] Erlinger TP, Tarver-Carr ME, Powe NR, Appel LJ, Coresh J, Eberhardt MS, and Brancati FL. Leukocytosis, hypoalbuminemia, and the risk for chronic kidney disease in US adults. *Am J Kidney Dis 42*: 256-263, 2003.

[29] Esposito BP, Breuer W, Slotki I, and Cabantchik ZI. Labile iron in parenteral iron formulations and its potential for generating plasma nontransferrin-bound iron in dialysis patients. *Eur J Clin Invest 32 Suppl 1*: 42-49, 2002.

[30] Fellstrom BC, Holdaas H, and Jardine AG. Why do we need a statin trial in hemodialysis patients? *Kidney Int Suppl:* S204-206, 2003.

[31] Fitzpatrick LA, Severson A, Edwards WD, and Ingram RT. Diffuse calcification in human coronary arteries. Association of osteopontin with atherosclerosis. *J Clin Invest 94*: 1597-1604, 1994.

[32] Fitzpatrick LA, Turner RT, and Ritman ER. Endochondral bone formation in the heart: a possible mechanism of coronary calcification. *Endocrinology 144*: 2214-2219, 2003.

[33] Fleck C, Schweitzer F, Karge E, Busch M, and Stein G. Serum concentrations of asymmetric (ADMA) and symmetric (SDMA) dimethylarginine in patients with chronic kidney diseases. *Clin Chim Acta 336*: 1-12, 2003.

[34] Fliser D, Kielstein JT, Haller H, and Bode-Boger SM. Asymmetric dimethylarginine: a cardiovascular risk factor in renal disease? *Kidney Int Suppl*: S37-40, 2003.

[35] Foley RN, Parfrey PS, and Sarnak MJ. Epidemiology of cardiovascular disease in chronic renal disease. *J Am Soc Nephrol 9*: S16-23, 1998.

[36] Fung F, Sherrard DJ, Gillen DL, Wong C, Kestenbaum B, Seliger S, Ball A, and Stehman-Breen C. Increased risk for cardiovascular mortality among malnourished end-stage renal disease patients. *Am J Kidney Dis 40*: 307-314, 2002.

[37] Galis ZS and Khatri JJ. Matrix metalloproteinases in vascular remodeling and atherogenesis: the good, the bad, and the ugly. *Circ Res 90*: 251-262, 2002.

[38] Girndt M, Kaul H, Sester U, Ulrich C, Sester M, Georg T, and Kohler H. Anti-inflammatory interleukin-10 genotype protects dialysis patients from cardiovascular events. *Kidney Int 62*: 949-955, 2002.

[39] Girndt M, Ulrich C, Kaul H, Sester U, Sester M, and Kohler H. Uremia-associated immune defect: the IL-10-CRP axis. *Kidney Int Suppl:* S76-79, 2003.

[40] Goodman WG, Goldin J, Kuizon BD, Yoon C, Gales B, Sider D, Wang Y, Chung J, Emerick A, Greaser L, Elashoff RM, and Salusky IB. Coronary-artery calcification in young adults with end-stage renal disease who are undergoing dialysis. *N Engl J Med 342:* 1478-1483, 2000.

[41] Guz G, Nurhan Ozdemir F, Sezer S, Isiklar I, Arat Z, Turan M, and Haberal M. Effect of apolipoprotein E polymorphism on serum lipid, lipoproteins, and atherosclerosis in hemodialysis patients. *Am J Kidney Dis 36*: 826-836, 2000.

[42] Harris KP, Wheeler DC, and Chong CC. A placebo-controlled trial examining atorvastatin in dyslipidemic patients undergoing CAPD. *Kidney Int 61*: 1469-1474, 2002.

[43] Haynes WG. Hyperhomocysteinemia, vascular function and atherosclerosis: effects of vitamins. *Cardiovasc Drugs Ther 16*: 391-399, 2002.

[44] Hilgendorff A, Muth H, Parviz B, Staubitz A, Haberbosch W, Tillmanns H, and Holschermann H. Statins differ in their ability to block NF-kappaB activation in human blood monocytes. *Int J Clin Pharmacol Ther 41*: 397-401, 2003.

[45] Himmelfarb J and McMonagle E. Albumin is the major plasma protein target of oxidant stress in uremia. *Kidney Int 60*: 358-363, 2001.

[46] Himmelfarb J, Stenvinkel P, Ikizler TA, and Hakim RM. The elephant in uremia: oxidant stress as a unifying concept of cardiovascular disease in uremia. *Kidney Int 62*: 1524-1538, 2002.

[47] Hojs R, Hojs-Fabjan T, and Balon BP. Atherosclerosis in patients with end-stage renal failure prior to initiation of hemodialysis. *Ren Fail 25*: 247-254, 2003.

[48] Huber SA, Sakkinen P, Conze D, Hardin N, and Tracy R. Interleukin-6 exacerbates early atherosclerosis in mice. *Arterioscler Thromb Vasc Biol 19*: 2364-2367, 1999.

[49] Hufnagel G, Michel C, Vrtovsnik F, Queffeulou G, Kossari N, and Mignon F. Effects of atorvastatin on dyslipidaemia in uraemic patients on peritoneal dialysis. *Nephrol Dial Transplant 15*: 684-688, 2000.

[50] Jadhav UM and Kadam NN. Association of microalbuminuria with carotid intima-media thickness and coronary artery disease--a cross-sectional study in Western India. *J Assoc Physicians India 50*: 1124-1129, 2002.

[51] Jadoul M, Ueda Y, Yasuda Y, Saito A, Robert A, Ishida N, Kurokawa K, Van Ypersele De Strihou C, and Miyata T. Influence of hemodialysis membrane type on pentosidine plasma level, a marker of "carbonyl stress". *Kidney Int 55*: 2487-2492, 1999.

[52] Jankowski J, van der Giet M, Jankowski V, Schmidt S, Hemeier M, Mahn B, Giebing G, Tolle M, Luftmann H, Schluter H, Zidek W, and Tepel M. Increased plasma phenylacetic acid in patients with end-stage renal failure inhibits iNOS expression. *J Clin Invest 112*: 256-264, 2003.

[53] Jungers P, Khoa TN, Massy ZA, Zingraff J, Labrunie M, Descamps-Latscha B, and Man NK. Incidence of atherosclerotic arterial occlusive accidents in predialysis and dialysis patients: a multicentric study in the Ile de France district. *Nephrol Dial Transplant 14*: 898-902, 1999.

[54] Jurkovitz CT, Abramson JL, Vaccarino LV, Weintraub WS, and McClellan WM. Association of high serum creatinine and anemia increases the risk of coronary events: results from the prospective community-based atherosclerosis risk in communities (ARIC) study. *J Am Soc Nephrol 14*: 2919-2925, 2003.

[55] Kalantar-Zadeh K, Ikizler TA, Block G, Avram MM, and Kopple JD. Malnutrition-inflammation complex syndrome in dialysis patients: Causes and consequences. *Am J Kidney Dis 42:* 864-881, 2003.

[56] Katzel LI, Fleg JL, Paidi M, Ragoobarsingh N, and Goldberg AP. ApoE4 polymorphism increases the risk for exercise-induced silent myocardial ischemia in older men. *Arterioscler Thromb 13*: 1495-1500, 1993.

[57] Kaysen GA. Role of inflammation and its treatment in ESRD patients. *Blood Purif 20*: 70-80, 2002.

[58] Ketteler M, Wanner C, Metzger T, Bongartz P, Westenfeld R, Gladziwa U, Schurgers LJ, Vermeer C, Jahnen-Dechent W, and Floege J. Deficiencies of calcium-regulatory proteins in dialysis patients: a novel concept of cardiovascular calcification in uremia. *Kidney Int Suppl*: S84-87, 2003.

[59] Kielstein JT, Bode-Boger SM, Frolich JC, Haller H, and Boger RH. Relationship of asymmetric dimethylarginine to dialysis treatment and atherosclerotic disease. *Kidney Int Suppl 78*: S9-13, 2001.

[60] Kielstein JT, Boger RH, Bode-Boger SM, Frolich JC, Haller H, Ritz E, and Fliser D. Marked increase of asymmetric dimethylarginine in patients with incipient primary chronic renal disease. *J Am Soc Nephrol 13*: 170-176, 2002.

[61] Kobayashi S, Moriya H, Aso K, and Ohtake T. Vitamin E-bonded hemodialyzer improves atherosclerosis associated with a rheological improvement of circulating red blood cells. *Kidney Int 63*: 1881-1887, 2003.
[62] Kone BC. Molecular biology of natriuretic peptides and nitric oxide synthases. *Cardiovasc Res 51*: 429-441, 2001.
[63] Kone BC. Nitric oxide in renal health and disease. *Am J Kidney Dis 30*: 311-333, 1997.
[64] Kone BC and Baylis C. Biosynthesis and homeostatic roles of nitric oxide in the normal kidney. *Am J Physiol 272*: F561-578, 1997.
[65] Lebreton JP, Joisel F, Raoult JP, Lannuzel B, Rogez JP, and Humbert G. Serum concentration of human alpha 2 HS glycoprotein during the inflammatory process: evidence that alpha 2 HS glycoprotein is a negative acute-phase reactant. *J Clin Invest 64:* 1118-1129, 1979.
[66] Leoncini G, Viazzi F, Parodi D, Vettoretti S, Ratto E, Ravera M, Tomolillo C, Del Sette M, Bezante GP, Deferrari G, and Pontremoli R. Mild renal dysfunction and subclinical cardiovascular damage in primary hypertension. *Hypertension 42*: 14-18, 2003.
[67] Libby P. Inflammation in atherosclerosis. *Nature 420:* 868-874, 2002.
[68] Lindner A, Charra B, Sherrard DJ, and Scribner BH. Accelerated Atherosclerosis in prolonged maintainance hemodialysis. *N Engl J Med 290*: 697-701, 1974.
[69] Locatelli F, Canaud B, Eckardt KU, Stenvinkel P, Wanner C, and Zoccali C. Oxidative stress in end-stage renal disease: an emerging threat to patient outcome. *Nephrol Dial Transplant 18:* 1272-1280, 2003.
[70] Locatelli F, Pozzoni P, Tentori F, and del Vecchio L. Epidemiology of cardiovascular risk in patients with chronic kidney disease. *Nephrol Dial Transplant 18 Suppl 7*: vii2-9, 2003.
[71] London GM, Guerin AP, Marchais SJ, Metivier F, Pannier B, and Adda H. Arterial media calcification in end-stage renal disease: impact on all-cause and cardiovascular mortality. *Nephrol Dial Transplant 18*: 1731-1740, 2003.
[72] London GM, Marchais SJ, Guerin AP, Metivier F, and Adda H. Arterial structure and function in end-stage renal disease. *Nephrol Dial Transplant 17*: 1713-1724, 2002.
[73] Lonn E, Yusuf S, Dzavik V, Doris C, Yi Q, Smith S, Moore-Cox A, Bosch J, Riley W, and Teo K. Effects of ramipril and vitamin E on atherosclerosis: the study to evaluate carotid ultrasound changes in patients treated with ramipril and vitamin E (SECURE). *Circulation 103*: 919-925, 2001.
[74] Loughrey CM, Young IS, Lightbody JH, McMaster D, McNamee PT, and Trimble ER. Oxidative stress in haemodialysis. *Qjm 87*: 679-683, 1994.
[75] Ludat K, Sommerburg O, Grune T, Siems WG, Riedel E, and Hampl H. Oxidation parameters in complete correction of renal anemia. *Clin Nephrol 53*: S30-35, 2000.
[76] Makita Z, Radoff S, Rayfield EJ, Yang Z, Skolnik E, Delaney V, Friedman EA, Cerami A, and Vlassara H. Advanced glycosylation end products in patients with diabetic nephropathy. *N Engl J Med 325*: 836-842, 1991.
[77] Mallat Z, Besnard S, Duriez M, Deleuze V, Emmanuel F, Bureau MF, Soubrier F, Esposito B, Duez H, Fievet C, Staels B, Duverger N, Scherman D, and Tedgui A. Protective role of interleukin-10 in atherosclerosis. *Circ Res 85*: e17-24, 1999.

[78] Merjanian R, Budoff M, Adler S, Berman N, and Mehrotra R. Coronary artery, aortic wall, and valvular calcification in nondialyzed individuals with type 2 diabetes and renal disease. *Kidney Int* 64: 263-271, 2003.

[79] Messerli AW, Seshadri N, Pearce GL, Sachar R, Hoogwerf BJ, and Sprecher DL. Relation of albumin/creatinine ratio to C-reactive protein and to the metabolic syndrome. *Am J Cardiol 92*: 610-612, 2003.

[80] Michelis R, Gery R, Sela S, Shurtz-Swirski R, Grinberg N, Snitkovski T, Shasha SM, and Kristal B. Carbonyl stress induced by intravenous iron during haemodialysis. *Nephrol Dial Transplant 18*: 924-930, 2003.

[81] Moe SM, O'Neill KD, Duan D, Ahmed S, Chen NX, Leapman SB, Fineberg N, and Kopecky K. Medial artery calcification in ESRD patients is associated with deposition of bone matrix proteins. *Kidney Int 61*: 638-647, 2002.

[82] Moeslinger T and Spieckermann PG. Urea-induced inducible nitric oxide synthase inhibition and macrophage proliferation. *Kidney Int Suppl 78*: S2-8, 2001.

[83] Moore KJ, Fitzgerald ML, and Freeman MW. Peroxisome proliferator-activated receptors in macrophage biology: friend or foe? *Curr Opin Lipidol 12*: 519-527, 2001.

[84] Moustapha A, Gupta A, Robinson K, Arheart K, Jacobsen DW, Schreiber MJ, and Dennis VW. Prevalence and determinants of hyperhomocysteinemia in hemodialysis and peritoneal dialysis. *Kidney Int 55*: 1470-1475, 1999.

[85] Moustapha A, Naso A, Nahlawi M, Gupta A, Arheart KL, Jacobsen DW, Robinson K, and Dennis VW. Prospective study of hyperhomocysteinemia as an adverse cardiovascular risk factor in end-stage renal disease. *Circulation 97*: 138-141, 1998.

[86] Muros M and Rodriguez-Ferrer C. Apolipoprotein E polymorphism influence on lipids, apolipoproteins and Lp(a) in a Spanish population underexpressing apo E4. *Atherosclerosis 121*: 13-21, 1996.

[87] Murtaugh MA, Jacobs DR, Jr., Yu X, Gross MD, and Steffes M. Correlates of urinary albumin excretion in young adult blacks and whites: the Coronary Artery Risk Development in Young Adults Study. *Am J Epidemiol 158*: 676-686, 2003.

[88] Naidoo DP. The link between microalbuminuria, endothelial dysfunction and cardiovascular disease in diabetes. *Cardiovasc J S Afr 13*: 194-199, 2002.

[89] Nishino T, Horii Y, Shiiki H, Yamamoto H, Makita Z, Bucala R, and Dohi K. Immunohistochemical detection of advanced glycosylation end products within the vascular lesions and glomeruli in diabetic nephropathy. *Hum Pathol 26*: 308-313, 1995.

[90] Ohkuma T, Minagawa T, Takada N, Ohno M, Oda H, and Ohashi H. C-reactive protein, lipoprotein(a), homocysteine, and male sex contribute to carotid atherosclerosis in peritoneal dialysis patients. *Am J Kidney Dis 42*: 355-361, 2003.

[91] Ortega O, Rodriguez I, Gallar P, Carreno A, Ortiz M, Espejo B, Jimenez J, Gutierrez M, Oliet A, and Vigil A. Significance of high C-reactive protein levels in pre-dialysis patients. *Nephrol Dial Transplant 17*: 1105-1109, 2002.

[92] Panichi V, Migliori M, De Pietro S, Taccola D, Bianchi AM, Norpoth M, Giovannini L, Palla R, and Tetta C. C-reactive protein as a marker of chronic inflammation in uremic patients. *Blood Purif 18*: 183-190, 2000.

[93] Pecoits-Filho R, Stenvinkel P, Marchlewska A, Heimburger O, Barany P, Hoff CM, Holmes CJ, Suliman M, Lindholm B, Schalling M, and Nordfors L. A functional variant of the myeloperoxidase gene is associated with cardiovascular disease in end-stage renal disease patients. *Kidney Int Suppl:* S172-176, 2003.
[94] Rattazzi M, Puato M, Faggin E, Bertipaglia B, Grego F, and Pauletto P. New markers of accelerated atherosclerosis in end-stage renal disease. *J Nephrol 16*: 11-20, 2003.
[95] Ravera M, Ratto E, Vettoretti S, Viazzi F, Leoncini G, Parodi D, Tomolillo C, Del Sette M, Maviglio N, Deferrari G, and Pontremoli R. Microalbuminuria and subclinical cerebrovascular damage in essential hypertension. *J Nephrol 15*: 519-524, 2002.
[96] Ridker PM, Cushman M, Stampfer MJ, Tracy RP, and Hennekens CH. Inflammation, aspirin, and the risk of cardiovascular disease in apparently healthy men. *N Engl J Med 336*: 973-979, 1997.
[97] Ridker PM, Hennekens CH, Buring JE, and Rifai N. C-reactive protein and other markers of inflammation in the prediction of cardiovascular disease in women. *N Engl J Med 342*: 836-843, 2000.
[98] Rosengren A, Wilhelmsen L, Eriksson E, Risberg B, and Wedel H. Lipoprotein (a) and coronary heart disease: a prospective case-control study in a general population sample of middle aged men. *Brit Med J 301*: 1248-1251, 1990.
[99] Ross R. Atherosclerosis--an inflammatory disease. *N Engl J Med 340*: 115-126, 1999.
[100] Sakata N, Imanaga Y, Meng J, Tachikawa Y, Takebayashi S, Nagai R, and Horiuchi S. Increased advanced glycation end products in atherosclerotic lesions of patients with end-stage renal disease. *Atherosclerosis 142*: 67-77, 1999.
[101] Saltissi D, Morgan C, Rigby RJ, and Westhuyzen J. Safety and efficacy of simvastatin in hypercholesterolemic patients undergoing chronic renal dialysis. *Am J Kidney Dis 39*: 283-290, 2002.
[102] Sarnak MJ and Levey AS. Cardiovascular disease and chronic renal disease: a new paradigm. *Am J Kidney Dis 35*: S117-131, 2000.
[103] Schmidt RJ, Yokota S, Tracy TS, Sorkin MI, and Baylis C. Nitric oxide production is low in end-stage renal disease patients on peritoneal dialysis. *Am J Physiol 276*: F794-797, 1999.
[104] Scholkens BA and Landgraf W. ACE inhibition and atherogenesis. *Can J Physiol Pharmacol 80:* 354-359, 2002.
[105] Schwarz U, Buzello M, Ritz E, Stein G, Raabe G, Wiest G, Mall G, and Amann K. Morphology of coronary atherosclerotic lesions in patients with end-stage renal failure. *Nephrol Dial Transplant 15*: 218-223, 2000.
[106] Schwedler S, Schinzel R, Vaith P, and Wanner C. Inflammation and advanced glycation end products in uremia: simple coexistence, potentiation or causal relationship? *Kidney Int Suppl 78*: S32-36, 2001.
[107] Schwedler SB, Metzger T, Schinzel R, and Wanner C. Advanced glycation end products and mortality in hemodialysis patients. *Kidney Int 62*: 301-310, 2002.
[108] Scribner AW, Loscalzo J, and Napoli C. The effect of angiotensin-converting enzyme inhibition on endothelial function and oxidant stress. *Eur J Pharmacol 482*: 95-99, 2003.

[109] Segura J, Campo C, and Ruilope LM. Proteinuria: an underappreciated risk factor in cardiovascular disease. *Curr Cardiol Rep 4:* 458-462, 2002.

[110] Seliger SL, Weiss NS, Gillen DL, Kestenbaum B, Ball A, Sherrard DJ, and Stehman-Breen CO. HMG-CoA reductase inhibitors are associated with reduced mortality in ESRD patients. *Kidney Int 61*: 297-304, 2002.

[111] Shanahan CM, Cary NR, Salisbury JR, Proudfoot D, Weissberg PL, and Edmonds ME. Medial localization of mineralization-regulating proteins in association with Monckeberg's sclerosis: evidence for smooth muscle cell-mediated vascular calcification. *Circulation 100:* 2168-2176, 1999.

[112] Shishehbor MH, Brennan ML, Aviles RJ, Fu X, Penn MS, Sprecher DL, and Hazen SL. Statins promote potent systemic antioxidant effects through specific inflammatory pathways. *Circulation 108*: 426-431, 2003.

[113] Shoji T, Emoto M, Tabata T, Kimoto E, Shinohara K, Maekawa K, Kawagishi T, Tahara H, Ishimura E, and Nishizawa Y. Advanced atherosclerosis in predialysis patients with chronic renal failure. *Kidney Int 61*: 2187-2192, 2002.

[114] Shoji T, Nishizawa Y, Kawagishi T, Kawasaki K, Taniwaki H, Tabata T, Inoue T, and Morii H. Intermediate-density lipoprotein as an independent risk factor for aortic atherosclerosis in hemodialysis patients. *J Am Soc Nephrol 9*: 1277-1284, 1998.

[115] Shoji T, Nishizawa Y, Kawagishi T, Tanaka M, Kawasaki K, Tabata T, Inoue T, and Morii H. Atherogenic lipoprotein changes in the absence of hyperlipidemia in patients with chronic renal failure treated by hemodialysis. *Atherosclerosis 131*: 229-236, 1997.

[116] Shulman NB, Ford CE, Hall WD, Blaufox MD, Simon D, Langford HG, and Schneider KA. Prognostic value of serum creatinine and effect of treatment of hypertension on renal function. Results from the hypertension detection and follow-up program. The Hypertension Detection and Follow-up Program Cooperative Group. *Hypertension 13:* I80-93, 1989.

[117] Sigurdsson G, Baldursdottir A, Sigvaldason H, Agnarsson U, Thorgeirsson G, and Sigfusson N. Predictive value of apolipoproteins in a prospective survey of coronary artery disease in men. *Am J Cardiol 69:* 1251-1254, 1992.

[118] Stam F, van Guldener C, Schalkwijk CG, ter Wee PM, Donker AJ, and Stehouwer CD. Impaired renal function is associated with markers of endothelial dysfunction and increased inflammatory activity. *Nephrol Dial Transplant 18*: 892-898, 2003.

[119] Stenvinkel P. Anaemia and inflammation: what are the implications for the nephrologist? *Nephrol Dial Transplant 18 Suppl 8: viii*17-22, 2003.

[120] Stenvinkel P. Inflammation in end-stage renal failure: could it be treated? *Nephrol Dial Transplant 17 Suppl 8*: 33-38; discussion 40, 2002.

[121] Stenvinkel P. The role of inflammation in the anaemia of end-stage renal disease. *Nephrol Dial Transplant 16 Suppl 7*: 36-40, 2001.

[122] Stenvinkel P, Andersson P, Wang T, Lindholm B, Bergstrom J, Palmblad J, Heimburger O, and Cederholm T. Do ACE-inhibitors suppress tumour necrosis factor-alpha production in advanced chronic renal failure? *J Intern Med 246*: 503-507, 1999.

[123] Stenvinkel P and Barany P. Anaemia, rHuEPO resistance, and cardiovascular disease in end-stage renal failure; links to inflammation and oxidative stress. *Nephrol Dial Transplant 17 Suppl 5*: 32-37, 2002.

[124] Stenvinkel P, Heimburger O, and Jogestrand T. Elevated interleukin-6 predicts progressive carotid artery atherosclerosis in dialysis patients: association with Chlamydia pneumoniae seropositivity. *Am J Kidney Dis 39*: 274-282, 2002.

[125] Stenvinkel P, Holmberg I, Heimburger O, and Diczfalusy U. A study of plasmalogen as an index of oxidative stress in patients with chronic renal failure. Evidence of increased oxidative stress in malnourished patients. *Nephrol Dial Transplant 13*: 2594-2600, 1998.

[126] Stenvinkel P, Pecoits-Filho R, and Lindholm B. Coronary artery disease in end-stage renal disease: no longer a simple plumbing problem. *J Am Soc Nephrol 14*: 1927-1939, 2003.

[127] Sukhova GK, Williams JK, and Libby P. Statins reduce inflammation in atheroma of nonhuman primates independent of effects on serum cholesterol. *Arterioscler Thromb Vasc Biol 22*: 1452-1458, 2002.

[128] Suliman ME, Stenvinkel P, Barany P, Heimburger O, Anderstam B, and Lindholm B. Hyperhomocysteinemia and its relationship to cardiovascular disease in ESRD: influence of hypoalbuminemia, malnutrition, inflammation, and diabetes mellitus. *Am J Kidney Dis 41*: S89-95, 2003.

[129] Sydor A, Drozdz M, Krasniak A, Milkowski A, Chmiel G, Malczak J, Zabawa-Holys S, Moskal K, Podwysocki A, Szmigielski M, Czarnecka D, Gozdecka H, Kowalczyk-Michalek M, Szczeklik A, Wiecek A, and Sulowicz W. [Hyperhomocysteinemia and advancement of atherosclerosis in patients with chronic renal failure on maintenance hemodialysis]. *Przegl Lek 59*: 962-967, 2002.

[130] Sydow K and Munzel T. ADMA and oxidative stress. *Atheroscler Suppl 4*: 41-51, 2003.

[131] Temelkova-Kurktschiev T, Koehler C, Henkel E, and Hanefeld M. Leukocyte count and fibrinogen are associated with carotid and femoral intima-media thickness in a risk population for diabetes. *Cardiovasc Res 56*: 277-283, 2002.

[132] Tepel M, van der Giet M, Statz M, Jankowski J, and Zidek W. The antioxidant acetylcysteine reduces cardiovascular events in patients with end-stage renal failure: a randomized, controlled trial. *Circulation 107*: 992-995, 2003.

[133] Tham DM, Martin-McNulty B, Wang YX, Wilson DW, Vergona R, Sullivan ME, Dole W, and Rutledge JC. Angiotensin II is associated with activation of NF-kappaB-mediated genes and downregulation of PPARs. *Physiol Genomics 11*: 21-30, 2002.

[134] Troxclair D, Boudreau DA, Malcom GT, Pedersen HS, Mulvad G, Newmann WP, 3rd, and Middaugh JP. Arterial calcification as a marker for atherosclerosis in three Arctic populations. *Int J Circumpolar Health 57 Suppl 1*: 306-311, 1998.

[135] Uhlig K, Levey AS, and Sarnak MJ. Traditional cardiac risk factors in individuals with chronic kidney disease. *Semin Dial 16*: 118-127, 2003.

[136] Vallance P, Leone A, Calver A, Collier J, and Moncada S. Accumulation of an endogenous inhibitor of nitric oxide synthesis in chronic renal failure. *Lancet 339*: 572-575, 1992.

[137] Wang AY, Wang M, Woo J, Lam CW, Li PK, Lui SF, and Sanderson JE. Cardiac valve calcification as an important predictor for all-cause mortality and cardiovascular

mortality in long-term peritoneal dialysis patients: a prospective study. *J Am Soc Nephrol 14*: 159-168, 2003.

[138] Wang AY, Woo J, Wang M, Sea MM, Ip R, Li PK, Lui SF, and Sanderson JE. Association of inflammation and malnutrition with cardiac valve calcification in continuous ambulatory peritoneal dialysis patients. *J Am Soc Nephrol 12*: 1927-1936, 2001.

[139] Wannamethee SG, Shaper AG, and Perry IJ. Serum creatinine concentration and risk of cardiovascular disease: a possible marker for increased risk of stroke. *Stroke 28*: 557-563, 1997.

[140] Wanner C and Krane V. Uremia-specific alterations in lipid metabolism. *Blood Purif 20:* 451-453, 2002.

[141] Yamamura T, Dong LM, and Yamamoto A. Apolipoprotein E polymorphism and coronary heart disease. *Chin Med J (Engl) 105*: 738-741, 1992.

[142] Yu Y, Hou F, Zhou H, Yang Y, Zhang X, Yang L, and Hu M. [The role of hyperhomocysteinemia on atherosclerosis in patients with chronic renal failure]. *Zhonghua Nei Ke Za Zhi 41*: 517-521, 2002.

[143] Zhang R, Brennan ML, Fu X, Aviles RJ, Pearce GL, Penn MS, Topol EJ, Sprecher DL, and Hazen SL. Association between myeloperoxidase levels and risk of coronary artery disease. *JAMA 286*: 2136-2142, 2001.

[144] Zimmerman MA, Selzman CH, Cothren C, Sorensen AC, Raeburn CD, and Harken AH. Diagnostic implications of C-reactive protein. *Arch Surg 138*: 220-224, 2003.

[145] Zoccali C, Benedetto FA, Maas R, Mallamaci F, Tripepi G, Malatino LS, and Boger R. Asymmetric dimethylarginine, C-reactive protein, and carotid intima-media thickness in end-stage renal disease. *J Am Soc Nephrol 13*: 490-496, 2002.

[146] Zoccali C, Bode-Boger S, Mallamaci F, Benedetto F, Tripepi G, Malatino L, Cataliotti A, Bellanuova I, Fermo I, Frolich J, and Boger R. Plasma concentration of asymmetrical dimethylarginine and mortality in patients with end-stage renal disease: a prospective study. *Lancet 358*: 2113-2117, 2001.

[147] Zoccali C, Mallamaci F, and Tripepi G. Inflammation and atherosclerosis in end-stage renal disease. *Blood Purif 21*: 29-36, 2003.

Acknowledgments

Work in the authors' laboratory is sponsored by National Institutes of Health grants RO1-DK50745, RO1-DK47981 P50 GM-38529, and T32-DK61929, a Department of Defense "T5" grant, and endowment funds from The James T. and Nancy B. Willerson Chair of The University of Texas Health Sciences Center at Houston.

In: Current Topics in Atherosclerosis Research
Editor: Yong J. Geng, pp. 133-145

ISBN 1-59454-428-X

Chapter VII

Ion Channels in Atherosclerosis

Shigeru Morishima and Yong-Jian Geng*
Texas Heart Institute-St. Luke's Episcopal Hospital and University of Texas Health Science Center at Houston, School of Medicine

Abstract

Altered expression and function of ion channels occur in myogenic or non-myogenic vascular cells (i.e., smooth muscle cells and endothelial cells, respectively) during the development of atherosclerosis. The vascular ion channels play a key role in regulation of vascular cell contractility and homeostasis. In response to neurous stimulation, calcium channels contribute to cross-membrane signaling and maintanence of the contractility of vascular smooth muscle cells. Potassium channels are sensitive to voltage changes and mechnical stress in endothelial cells. The performance of the two types of contraction, phasic and tonic, requires expression of fully functional ion channels, receptor binding, protein kinases, and phosphorylation of myosin. Disorders of these ion channels and down-stream events may lead to dysfunction of vascular wall, including the abnormalities of the muscle tones, initiation of the muscle contraction as well as maintainance of the contraction strength and duration. Pharmaceutic approaches have been employed to correct the abnormalities, and many of them are not yet very successful. Further investigation is needed to deleanate the potential mechanism behind the ion channel disorders during atherosclerogenesis.

Keywords: Atherosclerosis, Ion channels, Blood vessels, Contraction, Homeostasis; Hypercholesterolemia

---

* Correspondence concerning this article should be addressed to Yong-Jian Geng, MD, PhD, the Center for Cardiovascular Biology and Atherosclerosis Research, Department of Internal Medicine, Universithy of Texas Health Science Center at Houston, TX 77030. Email: yong-jian.geng@uth.tmc.edu

Introduction

A variety of ion channels exist in vascular cells, which are involved in the development of atherosclerosis in the muscular arteries. [1, 2] Many risk factors for atherosclerosis can alter expression and function of ion channels in the arterial smooth muscle with characteristic pathological changes under influence of inflammation [3-5] and hyperlipidemia [6-8]. The vascular ion channels play an important role in regulation of vascular cell contractility and homeostasis. Contraction of vascular smooth muscle cells (SMC) can be classified into two states; phasic and tonic contraction. The performance of the two types of contraction requires the presence of normal ion channels, receptor binding, protein kinases, and phosphorylation of myosin. Ion channels regulate the muscle tones, and are responsible for initiating the muscle contraction as well as for maintaining the contraction strength and duration. Activation of ion channels results in changes in cross-plasma membrane action potentials, thus determining the tonic strength and sensitivity of myocytes to other stimulating factors. Although many types of ion channels may play roles in regulation of vascular SMC function, the channels for calcium, potassium and sodium are most interesting and extensively investigated. Ca^{2+} channels and ryanodine receptor channel, as well as Ca^{2+} pumps and Na-Ca exchanger, play also very important in determining intracellular Ca^{2+} level, which enhances the phosphorylation level of myosin and smooth muscle contraction. Recent investigations have shown that different types of ion channels contribute to atherosclerosis-triggered arterial spasm, a major cause of impaired blood flow. Abnormalities of ion channels may induce the imbalance of intracellular ionic homeostasis persistently, and thus augment muscle tonic strength. Many ion channels can alter behaviors of vascular cells, including their growth, proliferation, differentiation and death. In this chapter, we will review recent advances in ion channel research in atherosclerosis-related cardiovascular disease.

Ion Channels in Vascular Cells of Atherosclerotic Arteries

Ion channels expression and function in vascular smooth muscle cells and endothelial cells are known to play regulatory roles in vascular contraction and signal transduction. Many atheropathogenic factors may alter the ion channel function and subsequently trigger pathophysiological changes in the vessel wall. Different types of channels exist in vascular cells, including both muscle cells (i.e. smooth muscle cells or SMC) and non-muscle cells (i.e. endothelial cells or EC). Overall, the following types of ion channels function in regulation of a variety of cell bioactivities.

Calcium Release from Sarcoplasmic Reticulum

Activation of G protein-coupled receptors, such as those for α-adrenergics, muscarinics, prostaglandin $F_{2\alpha}$, angitotensin II or endothelin-1, results in activation of phospholipase C (PLC) and the phosphodiesteric breakdown of the phosphatidyl inositol 4,5-bisphosphate (PIP_2) into inositol 1,4,5-trisphosphate (IP_3) and 1,2-diacylglycerol (DAG). IP_3 causes a release of Ca^{2+} from the sarcoplasmic reticulum (SR) through IP3 receptor channel in smooth muscle. The released intracellular Ca^{2+} binds to calmodulin (CaM), and the Ca^{2+}-CaM complex activates myosin light chain kinase (MLCK). MLCK causes the smooth muscle to contract by the phosphorylation myosin light chain (MLC). This is the major signaling pathway for smooth muscle contraction. Cox et al. reported [9] the effects of dietary atherosclerosis on the pharmacology and ion channel properties of rabbit portal vein (PV). New Zealand White rabbits were fed normal rabbit chow +/- 2% cholesterol for 10 wk. Contractions to norepinephrine (NE) and serotonin were studied under isometric conditions with longitudinal strips. Ca^{2+} and K^+ currents (ICa and IK, respectively) were recorded in freshly dispersed myocytes by whole cell voltage clamp methods. Cholesterol feeding increased total plasma cholesterol levels from 28.4 +/- 5.2 to 1,387 +/- 172 mg/dl as well as the cholesterol-to-phospholipid molar ratio of the PV from 0.34 +/- 0.02 to 0.66 +/- 0.08. Only maximum contractile responses to serotonin were larger in atherosclerotic PV when normalized to the maximum KCl response. Concentration-active stress curves of the atherosclerotic PV to NE and serotonin were shifted to the left. Maximum values of ICa were larger in myocytes from atherosclerotic compared with control animals (4.4 +/- 0.4 vs. 3.1 +/- 0.2 pA/pF, $P < 0.05$). The voltage dependence of activation and availability of ICa was shifted toward more negative potentials by approximately 10 mV. Whole cell K^+ currents were smaller in atherosclerotic myocytes. At a test voltage of +20 mV, IK averaged 14.9 +/- 2.8 pA/pF in control compared with 7.7 +/- 0.8 pA/pF in atherosclerotic myocytes from a holding potential of -80 mV with external Ca^{2+} concentration of 5 mM. The reversal potential for IK tail currents was significantly less negative in atherosclerotic myocytes (-70 +/- 1 vs. -64 +/- 1 mV). These results suggest that atherosclerosis may have a negative impact on the ion channels of SR.

Store(receptor)-Operated Calcium Entry

When calcium store in sarcoplasmic reticulum is depleted or reduced, IP3 receptor channel induces extracellular Ca^{2+} to enter the cell through a plama membrane ion channel, TRPC1. There is a physical association between IP3R and TRPC1 crosslinked with another protein Homer. The increase of intracellular calcium by TRPC1 channel is known not only to refill Ca^{2+} into the store, but also to augment the muscle contraction. Loss of the smooth muscle contractile phenotype is critical in atherosclerosis and in restenosis after angioplasty, but its early signals are incompletely understood. Recent studies[10] have provided evidence supporting the role of transient receptor potential canonical (TRPC) proteins, which have been suggested to mediate store-operated Ca^{2+} entry (SOCE). Contractility of rat cerebral arteries in organ culture is preserved for several days, whereas SOCE is increased. In correlation with this increase is that nifedipine-insensitive whole cell current, activated by depletion of intracellular Ca^{2+} stores, was increased by 50% in cells isolated from arteries cultured for 3 days. Bergdahl, et al. performed in vitro studies showing that TRPC1 and TRPC6 mRNA were more than fivefold increased in cells isolated after organ culture, whereas TRPC3 was decreased. Immunofluorescent staining and/or Western blotting of arteries and isolated cells showed upregulation of TRPC1 and TRPC6 proteins during organ culture. In intact arteries, TRPC4 expression correlated with the amount of endothelium present. Ca^{2+} addition after store depletion caused a contraction in cultured, but not in freshly dissected, arteries. A polyclonal TRPC1 antibody directed against an extracellular epitope inhibited this contraction by approximately 50%. To investigate the basis of the TRPC upregulation and assess its possible clinical significance, segments of human internal mammary artery were organ cultured for 24 h and then exposed to balloon dilatation in vitro, followed by further culturing for up to 48 h. After dilatation, TRPC1 and TRPC6 mRNA were progressively increased compared with undilated control segments. The results of this study indicate that vascular injury enhances plasticity in TRPC expression, that TRPC expression correlates with cellular Ca^{2+} handling, and that TRPC1 is a subunit of upregulated store-operated Ca^{2+} channels.

Voltage-Dependent Channels

Another main pathway of calcium entry is mediated by voltage-dependent Ca channels. Voltage-dependent Ca channels in smooth muscle cells are L-type, a high-voltage activated calcium channel, and T-type, a low-voltage activated calcium channel. The entry through these channels induces release of Ca^{2+} from SR. The channel on SR membrane is inhibited by ryanodine, and different from IP3R. This ryanodine receptor channel releases SR-stored calcium mostly when calcium enters through voltage-dependent calcium channels (calcium-induced calcium release). Hypercholesterolemia serves as a primary risk factor for the development of coronary heart disease. Coronary ion regulation, especially calcium, is thought to be important in coronary heart disease development. There is evidence that high dietary fat and cholesterol affects coronary arterial smooth muscle (CASM) ion channels mainly in large arteries. Bowles, et al. [6] conducted experiments to determine the effect of diet-induced HC on CASM voltage-gated calcium current (I(Ca)). They fed male miniature swine a high-fat, high-cholesterol diet (40% kcal fat, 2% wt cholesterol) for 20-24 wk, which resulted in elevated serum total and low-density lipoprotein cholesterol. Histochemistry indicated early atherosclerosis in large coronary arteries. CASM were isolated from the right coronary artery (>1.0 mm ID), small arteries (approximately 200 microm), and large arterioles (approximately 100 microm). I(Ca) was determined by whole cell voltage clamp. L-type I(Ca) was reduced approximately 30% by HC compared with controls in the right coronary artery (-5.29 +/- 0.42 vs. -7.59 +/- 0.41 pA/pF) but not the microcirculation (small artery, -8.39 +/- 0.80 vs. -10.13 +/- 0.60; arterioles, -10.78 +/- 0.93 vs. -11.31 +/- 0.95 pA/pF). Voltage-dependent activation was unaffected by HC in both the macro- and microcirculation. L-type voltage-gated calcium channel (Ca(v)1.2) mRNA and membrane protein levels were unaffected by HC. Inhibition of I(Ca) by HC was reversed in vitro by the cholesterol scavenger methyl-beta-cyclodextrin and mimicked in control CASM by incubation with the cholesterol donor cholesterol:methyl-beta-cyclodextrin. These data indicate that CASM L-type I(Ca) is decreased in large coronary arteries in early stages of atherosclerosis, whereas I(Ca) in the microcirculation is unaffected. The inhibition of calcium channel activity in CASM of large coronary arteries is likely due to increases in membrane free cholesterol.

Voltage-gated, delayed rectifier K^+ current (KV) that is sensitive to 4-aminopyridine (4AP) block has been identified in vascular smooth muscle tissues. [11] These channels conduct outward, hyperpolarizing K^+ current that influences resting membrane potential and contributes to repolarization of action potentials. Smooth muscle cells in most arterial resistance vessels regulate Ca^{2+} influx and contractile tone by low amplitude, tonic changes in membrane potential. Block of KV with 4-aminopyridine leads to contraction and an enhanced myogenic response to increased intravascular pressure. Cole, at al. [11] investigated the modulation of KV currents in isolated, freshly dispersed smooth muscle cells from rabbit portal vein and coronary arteries in whole-cell voltage clamp experiments. Our findings indicate that KV channels are regulated by signal transduction mechanisms involving vasoactive agonists that activate cAMP-dependent protein kinase (PKA) or protein kinase C (PKC). The properties and potential function of KV channels in vascular smooth muscle are closely associated with beta-adrenoceptors, adenylyl cyclase and PKA, as well as angiotensin system, diacylglycerol, and PKC.

Stretch-Activated Channels

Several ion channels present in vascular cells are responsible for mechanic stimulation from blood flow and pressure. [12, 13] The channels promptly open when the cellular plasma membrane is mechanically stretched. Hence, they serve as a biological sensor to mechanic force. Some of the stretch-activated ion channels can permeate Ca^{2+}, while others may be K^+ channels. The stretch-activated ion channels exist prominently in vascular ECs and SMCs, as they are always exposed to hemodynamic forces, such as fluid shear stress. Compared to SMCs, vascular ECs seem more distinguished among and respond differently to different types of fluid mechanical shear stress. Elucidating the mechanisms governing this differential responsiveness is the key to understanding why early atherosclerotic lesions localize preferentially in arterial regions exposed to low and/or oscillatory flow. An early and very rapid endothelial response to flow is the activation of flow-sensitive K^+ and Cl(-) channels that respectively hyperpolarize and depolarize the cell membrane and regulate several important endothelial responses to flow. Lieu at al. [12] have used whole cell current- and voltage-clamp techniques to demonstrate that flow-sensitive hyperpolarizing and depolarizing currents respond differently to different types of shear stress in cultured bovine aortic ECs. They found that a steady shear stress level of 10 dyn/cm(2) activated both currents leading to rapid membrane hyperpolarization that was subsequently reversed to depolarization. In contrast, a steady shear stress of 1 dyn/cm(2) only activated the hyperpolarizing current. A purely oscillatory shear stress of 0 +/- 10 dyn/cm(2) with an oscillation frequency of either 1 or 0.2 Hz activated the hyperpolarizing current but only minimally the depolarizing current, whereas a 5-Hz oscillation activated neither current. These results demonstrate for the first time that flow-activated ion currents exhibit different sensitivities to shear stress magnitude and oscillation frequency. It is likely that flow-sensitive ion channels constitute components of an integrated mechanosensing system that, through the aggregate effect of ion channel activation on cell membrane potential, enables ECs to distinguish among different types of flow.

Steady laminar shear stress has been shown previously to markedly increase Na-K-Cl cotransporter mRNA and protein in human umbilical vein endothelial cells and also to rapidly increase endothelial K^+ and Cl(-) channel conductances. The effects of shear stress on Na-K-Cl cotransporter activity and protein expression in bovine aortic endothelial cells (BAEC) may be dependent on early changes in K^+ and Cl(-) channel conductances. Suvatne et al. [13] exposed confluent BAEC monolayers in a parallel-plate flow chamber to either steady shear stress (19 dyn/cm(2)) or purely oscillatory shear stress (0 +/- 19 dyn/cm(2)) for 6-48 h. They found that steady shear stress led to a 2- to 4-fold increase in BAEC cotransporter protein levels and a 1.5- to 1.8-fold increase in cotransporter activity, increases that were sustained over the longest time periods studied. Oscillatory flow, in contrast, had no effect on cotransporter protein levels. In the presence of flow-sensitive K^+ and Cl(-) channel pharmacological blockers, the steady shear stress-induced increase in cotransporter protein was virtually abolished. These results suggest that shear stress modulates the expression of the BAEC Na-K-Cl cotransporter by mechanisms that are dependent on flow-activated ion channels.

Other Factors for Maintenance of Intracellular Calcium Level

Calcium pumps both on plasma and sarcoplasmic membrane triggers efflux of Ca^{2+} and decrease cytoplasmic Ca^{2+}. The pumps are ATP-dependent, and when ATP exhausts under certain pathological conditions, such as ischemia, the pumps stop working. This is one of the important mechanisms leading to the calcium overloading under ischemic or hypoxia stress. DAG, a byproduct by PLC, activates protein kinase C (PKC), which can also enhance the phosphorylation of MLC and the contraction of smooth muscle. In addition, recently oxygen radicals have been reported to play a critical role in activation of some the channels or channel-associated kinase activities. For instance, hydrogen peroxide (H_2O_2) and reactive oxygen species implicated in inflammation, ischemia-reperfusion injury, and atherosclerosis, have impacts on the functions of ion channels. Bychkow et al. [5] showed that as recorded for K^+ currents and membrane potential by voltage- and current-clamp techniques, treatment with H_2O_2 elicited both hyperpolarization and depolarization of the membrane potential in a concentration-dependent manner. Low H_2O_2 concentrations (0.01 to 0.25 micromol/L) inhibited the inward-rectifying K^+ current (KIR). Whole-cell K^+ current analysis revealed that H_2O_2 (1 mmol/L) applied to the bath solution increased the Ca2+-dependent K^+ current (KCa) amplitude. H_2O_2 increased KCa current in outside-out patches in a Ca2+-free solution. When catalase (5000 micro/mL) was added to the bath solution, the outward-rectifying K^+ current amplitude was restored. In contrast, superoxide dismutase (1000 u/mL) had only a small effect on the H_2O_2-induced K^+ current changes. Next, we measured whole-cell K^+ currents and redox potentials simultaneously with a novel redox potential-sensitive electrode. The H_2O_2-mediated KCa current increase was accompanied by a whole-cell redox potential decrease. Thus, H_2O_2 elicited both hyperpolarization and depolarization of the membrane potential through 2 different mechanisms. Low H_2O_2 concentrations inhibited inward-rectifying K^+ currents, whereas higher H_2O_2 concentrations increased the amplitude of the outward K^+ current.

Channel Antagonists and Therapy for Atherosclerosis

Extensive research has been conducted for last several decades to establish the relationship between the high calcium level and the development of vascular diseases in particular atherosclerosis and hypertension. [14, 15] Since hypertension is one of the major risk factor of atherosclerotic coronary heart disease, the calcium loading in SMC with hypertension is primarily interesting. It is still controversial as to whether high dietary uptake or elevated serum calcium level causes hypertension. Certain dihydropyridine calcium channel blockers (CCBs) inhibit atherosclerotic lesion formation both in animal models and in human studies. Treatment with high dosages of certain dihydropyridine CCBs can significantly reduce atherosclerotic lesion development in cholersterol-fed rabbits [14]. In human study, amlodipine therapy is also associated with significant reduction in carotid atherosclerosis independently of blood pressure changes. Although the exact mechanism is still under investigation, CCBs are known to work through several potential mechanisms, which may or may not be independent of its antihypertensive effect.

The initial molecular and cellular events in atherogenesis are triggered by endothelial dysfunction, resulting in inflammation. In this early inflammatory response to atherosclerosis, the release of cytokines from the diseased vessel and other peripheral sites leads to the accumulation of mononuclear cells, migration and proliferation of smooth muscle cells that eventually results in the formation of the mature atherosclerotic plaque. As a number of these cellular and inflammatory processes are mediated by disruption in calcium homeostasis, there has been interest in the potential role of CCBs as antiatherogenic agents. This hypothesis has been extensively tested in a variety of cellular and animal models of atherosclerosis. Smooth muscle cells and macrophages, which synthesize matrix products and accumulate intracellular lipids, play a central role in lesion formation. Smooth muscle cell hyperplasia, with intracellular and functional changes, is common to both atherosclerosis and hypertension. The antiatherogenic properties of CCBs may be related in part to the protection of arterial cells from calcium overload through inhibition of calcium flux across voltage-regulated ion channels. Also, Ca^{2+} store in SR of genetically hypertensive rats was reported to be higher than normotensive rats.

CCBs may inhibit atherosclerotic lesion formation in rabbit models by reduction of calcium, lipid, and matrix accumulation in the arterial wall. [2] The mechanisms of these antiatherogenic effects are under investigation. Smooth muscle cells and macrophages, which synthesize matrix products and accumulate intracellular lipids, play a central role in lesion formation. Smooth muscle cell hyperplasia, with intracellular and functional changes, is common to both atherosclerosis and hypertension. The antiatherogenic properties of CCBs may be related in part to the protection of arterial cells from calcium overload through inhibition of calcium flux across voltage-regulated ion channels. CCBs may also inhibit cell migration, influence the uptake and catabolism of lipoproteins, alter smooth muscle matrix synthesis, and promote the depletion of intracellular cholesteryl ester stores. It appears that CCBs may inhibit the development of atherosclerotic lesions by two sets of mechanisms: alteration of lipid metabolism in smooth muscle cells and regulation of calcium-initiated or -accelerated intracellular processes.

VASORELAXATION, INFLAMMATION AND APOPTOSIS

Endothelial Cell Function

Blood flow interactions with the vascular endothelium represent a specialized example of mechanical regulation of cell function that has important physiological and pathological cardiovascular consequences. The endothelial monolayer in vivo acts as a signal transduction interface for forces associated with flowing blood (hemodynamic forces) in the acute regulation of artery tone and chronic structural remodeling of arteries, including the pathology of atherosclerosis. Mechanisms related to spatial relationships at the cell surfaces and throughout the cell that influence flow-mediated endothelial mechanotransduction are discussed. In particular, flow-mediated ion channel activation and cytoskeletal dynamics are considered in relation to topographic analyses of the luminal and abluminal surfaces of living endothelial cells.[16, 17] Vasoconstriction and the compromised ability of an artery to dilate are likely consequences of defective K^+ channel function in blood vessels during these disease states. In some instances, increased K^+ channel function may help to compensate for increased vascular tone. Endothelial cell dysfunction is commonly associated with cardiovascular disease, and altered activity of nitric oxide, prostacyclin, and endothelium-derived hyperpolarizing factor could also contribute to changes in resting K^+ channel activity, E(m), and K^+ channel-mediated vasodilatation. The current knowledge concerning the effects of disease on vascular K^+ channel function almost exclusively relies on interpretation of data obtained by using pharmacological modulators of K^+ channels [1]. As further progress is made in the development of more selective drugs and through molecular approaches such as gene targeting technology in mice, specific K^+ channel abnormalities and their causes in particular diseases should be more readily identified, providing novel directions for vascular therapy.

A variety of potassium channels exist on membranes of excitable cells. Most cells contain higher levels of intracellular potassium against that in the extracellular microenvironment. Consequently, the equilibrium potential of potassium is in the range of –100 to –70 mV, which means resting membrane potential of cells will be in that range when they have only potassium conductance. It matches that found in cardiomyocytes and many neurons whose resting membrane potential is around –80 mV. Having comparatively high potassium conductance in their resting state, SMCs gained the resting membrane potential of –35 to –60 mV, suggesting that the cells have other ion channel conductance, and that their membrane potential may become higher, if more potassium channels open. Additionally, in smooth muscle cells, as well as most excitable cells, potassium channels are involved in the repolarization phase of their action potential followed by depolarization by voltage-gated sodium channel.

Vascular Smooth Muscle Function

Potassium ion (K^+) channel activity acts as a major regulator of vascular muscle cell membrane potential (E_m), and therefore an important determinant of vascular tone. There is growing evidence that the function of several types of vascular K^+ channels is altered during major cardiovascular diseases, such as chronic hypertension, diabetes, and atherosclerosis [1]. Potassium channels are mainly classified by their gating machnism and molecular structure: voltage-gated (Kv), inward-rectifying (Kir), and calcium-activated (K_{Ca}) potassium channels. Calcium-activated potassium channels and ATP-regulated potassium channel play most important roles in regulating muscle tone in vascular smooth muscle cells. As intracellular calcium rises, K_{Ca} channels are activated, followed by membrane repolarization or sometimes, hyperpolarization of SMC mebrane due to the outward K current through the channels. ATP-dependent potassium channel is a unique channel whose openings are directly regulated by amount of ATP. When intracellular ATP decreases, K_{ATP} is activated and SMC resting membrane potential is hyperpolarized. Reagents which can open K_{ATP} channel have been developed. These potassium channel openers, such as cromakalim or nicorandil, can hyperpolarize the resting potential of SMCs, and relax muscle tone in the same mechniasm as that of K_{Ca} channel. These potassium channels have been known to have anti-atherosclerotic effect. The main mechanism of the effect is suggested to that these channels can reduce the tone of smooth muscle, thus hypertrophy through MAPK system and intracellular Ca overload would be suppressed. A report showed that free radials were decreased by a potassium channel opener levcromakalim. On the other hand, it is reported that relaxation of atherosclerotic arteries may be impaired during activation of K_{ATP}. KATP channel is notable for its cell-protective characteristics. Mitochondrial, but not plasmalemmal, subtype of KATP channel is well studied related to ischemic preconditioning in cardiomocytes. Studies showed the protective effect of ischemic preconditioning is mediated by KATP channel opening followed by PKC activation. The blockade of KATP channel opening abolishes almost all PKC-mediated cell-protective effects on ischemic cardiomyocytes.

It is not known if this channel has its protective effect on vascular SMCs or endothelial cells. In an experimental model, Pongo et al. [7] found that the protein kinase C-K(ATP) channel pathway was deteriorated in hypercholesterolaemic rabbits. They studied the effect of experimental hypercholesterolaemia/atherosclerosis on changes in coronary flow and cardiac function, induced by protein kinase C and ATP-sensitive K^+ (K(ATP)) channel modulators in isolated Langendorff-perfused rabbit hearts. Both phorbol 12-myristate-13-acetate (PMA) and phorbol 12,13-dibutyrate (PDB, 0.1 microM each), activators of protein kinase C, decreased, whereas staurosporine, (0.1 microM), a protein kinase C inhibitor, increased coronary flow and left ventricular dP/dt, an index of ventricular contractility. Glyburide (5-50 microM), a K(ATP) channel inhibitor, blocked the effect of staurosporine.

The phorbol esters were without effect in the presence of pinacidil (5 microM), a K(ATP) channel activator. Neither the protein kinase C modulators nor glyburide produced any effect on coronary flow and left ventricular contractility, when the hearts were prepared from animals either maintained on a cholesterol (1.5%)-enriched diet or treated with lovastatin (5 mg/kg/day per os). Treatment with farnesol (1 mg/kg twice a day for 7 days intravenously) restored the reactivity of hearts from either hypercholesterolaemic or lovastatin-treated animals to protein kinase C modulators. This study concludes that non-cholesterol mevalonate products are necessary for the functional integrity of the protein kinase C-K(ATP) channel pathway in the rabbit heart.

Inflammation

Atherosclerosis has been recognized as a chronic inflammatory disease. Amlodipine (a new class of calcium channel antagonist) has been shown to limit the progression of arteriosclerosis and decrease the incidence of cardiovascular events. Kataoka, et al.[3] have recently demonstrated that amlodipine attenuates the development of arteriosclerosis through the inhibition of inflammation in vivo. Long-term inhibition of nitric oxide (NO) by administration of a NO synthase inhibitor, N(omega)-nitro-L-arginine methyl ester (L-NAME), to rats induces coronary vascular inflammation [monocyte infiltration, monocyte chemoattractant protein-1 (MCP-1) expression, increased activity of angiotensin-converting enzyme (ACE)], and arteriosclerosis. Here, we used the rat model to investigate the anti-inflammatory effects of amlodipine in vivo. Treatment with amlodipine markedly inhibited the L-NAME-induced increase in vascular inflammation, oxidative stress, and local ACE and Rho activity and prevented arteriosclerosis. Interestingly, amlodipine prevented the L-NAME-induced increase in MCP-1 receptor CCR2 expression in circulating monocytes. Amlodipine markedly attenuated the high mortality rate at 8 wk of treatment. These data suggest that amlodipine attenuated arteriosclerosis through inhibiting inflammatory disorders in the rat model of long-term inhibition of NO synthesis. The anti-inflammatory effects of amlodipine seem to be mediated not only by the inhibition of local factors such as MCP-1 but also by the decrease in CCR2 in circulating monocytes. Inhibition of the MCP-1 to CCR2 pathway may represent novel anti-inflammatory actions of amlodipine beyond blood pressure lowering. In the rat endotoxic model, Chou, et al. [4] showed that the serum nitrite/nitrate, TNF-alpha and IL-1beta levels as well as iNOS protein expression of lungs were also suppressed by administration of amlodipine (50 microg/kg, i.v.). These results suggest that amlodipine may exert vascular beneficial effects by suppressing pro-inflammatory cytokines and free radical generation as well as iNOS induction in smooth muscle cells during activation of inflammatory mechanism. Thus, this channel blocker can exert anti-inflammatory effects on vascular cells.

Apoptosis

Restoration of cell volume after cell swelling in mammalian cells is achieved by the loss of solutes (K^+, Cl^-, and organic osmolytes) and the subsequent osmotically driven efflux of water. This process is generally known as regulatory volume decrease (RVD). [18] One pathway for the swelling induced loss of Cl- (and also organic osmolytes) during RVD is the volume-regulated anion channel (VRAC). VRAC is more than a volume regulator and that it participates in other fundamental cellular processes such as cell proliferation and apoptosis. The second part concentrates on the Rho/Rho kinase/myosin phosphorylation cascade and on compartmentalization in caveolae as modulators of the signal transduction cascade that controls VRAC gating in vascular endothelial cells. Intracellular K^+ plays an important role in controlling the cytoplasmic ion homeostasis for maintaining cell volume and inhibiting apoptotic enzymes in the cytosol and nucleus. Cytoplasmic K^+ concentration is mainly regulated by K^+ uptake via Na^+-K^+-ATPase and K^+ efflux through K^+ channels in the plasma membrane. Carbonyl cyanide p-trifluoromethoxyphenylhydrazone (FCCP), a protonophore that dissipates the H^+ gradient across the inner membrane of mitochondria, induces apoptosis in many cell types. [19] In rat and human pulmonary artery smooth muscle cells (PASMC), FCCP opens the large-conductance, voltage- and Ca2+-sensitive K^+ (maxi-K) channels, increased K^+ currents through maxi-K channels [I(K(Ca))], and induced apoptosis. Tetraethylammonia (1 mM) and iberiotoxin (100 nM) can decrease I(K(Ca)) by blocking the sarcolemmal maxi-K channels and inhibit the FCCP-induced apoptosis in PASMC cultured in media containing serum and growth factors. Furthermore, inhibition of K^+ efflux by raising extracellular K^+ concentration from 5 to 40 mM also attenuates PASMC apoptosis induced by FCCP and the K^+ ionophore valinomycin. [19] Hence, FCCP-mediated apoptosis in PASMC is partially due to an increase of maxi-K channel activity. The resultant K^+ loss through opened maxi-K channels may serve as a trigger for cell shrinkage and caspase activation.

Summary

Ion channels play a very important role in regulation of functions of vascular cells of arteries with or without atherosclerosis. Regardless of the causes that induce atherogenesis, expression and function of certain ion channels are altered in vascular cells during the development of atherosclerosis. Although many other types of ion channels are involved in the alterations in vascular cell function, the channels participating in cross-membrane signaling, stress response, and contractility seem to play central roles in regulation of vascular cell function and response to atherogenic stimulation. It is not completely understood about the mechanisms for the involvement of ion channels. They are mainly classified into two aspects: one is their effect on the contractile activity in smooth muscle cells, and the other is their homeostatic and cell-protective functions universally found in all types of cells. Voltage-dependent calcium channels and some potassium channels are known to be involved in regulating vascular tone, smooth muscle cell contraction, proliferation of many types of cells, and cell-protective function.

REFERENCES

[1] Sobey, CG. Potassium channel function in vascular disease. *Arterioscler Thromb Vasc Biol* 21(1):28-38,2001.

[2] Sowers, JR. Calcium channel blockers and atherosclerosis. *Am J Kidney Dis* 16(4 Suppl 1):3-9,1990.

[3] Kataoka, C, K Egashira, M Ishibashi, S Inoue, W Ni, K Hiasa, S Kitamoto, M Usui, and A Takeshita. Novel anti-inflammatory actions of amlodipine in a rat model of arteriosclerosis induced by long-term inhibition of nitric oxide synthesis. *Am J Physiol Heart Circ Physiol* 286(2):H768-74,2004.

[4] Chou, TC, SP Yang, and D Pei. Amlodipine inhibits pro-inflammatory cytokines and free radical production and inducible nitric oxide synthase expression in lipopolysaccharide/interferon-gamma-stimulated cultured vascular smooth muscle cells. *Jpn J Pharmacol* 89(2):157-63,2002.

[5] Bychkov, R, K Pieper, C Ried, M Milosheva, E Bychkov, FC Luft, and H Haller. Hydrogen peroxide, potassium currents, and membrane potential in human endothelial cells. *Circulation* 99(13):1719-25,1999.

[6] Bowles, DK, CL Heaps, JR Turk, KK Maddali, and EM Price. Hypercholesterolemia inhibits L-type calcium current in coronary macro-, not microcirculation. *J Appl Physiol* 96(6):2240-8,2004.

[7] Pongo, E, Z Balla, K Mubagwa, W Flameng, I Edes, Z Szilvassy, and P Ferdinandy. Deterioration of the protein kinase C-K(ATP) channel pathway in regulation of coronary flow in hypercholesterolaemic rabbits. *Eur J Pharmacol* 418(3):217-23,2001.

[8] Abrams, J. Clinical practice. Chronic stable angina. *N Engl J Med* 352(24):2524-33,2005.

[9] Cox, RH and TN Tulenko. Altered contractile and ion channel function in rabbit portal vein with dietary atherosclerosis. *Am J Physiol* 268(6 Pt 2):H2522-30,1995.

[10] Bergdahl, A, MF Gomez, AK Wihlborg, D Erlinge, A Eyjolfson, SZ Xu, DJ Beech, K Dreja, and P Hellstrand. Plasticity of TRPC expression in arterial smooth muscle: correlation with store-operated Ca^{2+} entry. *Am J Physiol Cell Physiol* 288(4):C872-80,2005.

[11] Cole, WC, O Clement-Chomienne, and EA Aiello. Regulation of 4-aminopyridine-sensitive, delayed rectifier K^+ channels in vascular smooth muscle by phosphorylation. *Biochem Cell Biol* 74(4):439-47,1996.

[12] Lieu, DK, PA Pappone, and AI Barakat. Differential membrane potential and ion current responses to different types of shear stress in vascular endothelial cells. *Am J Physiol Cell Physiol* 286(6):C1367-75,2004.

[13] Suvatne, J, AI Barakat, and ME O'Donnell. Flow-induced expression of endothelial Na-K-Cl cotransport: dependence on K^+ and Cl^- channels. *Am J Physiol Cell Physiol* 280(1):C216-27,2001.

[14] Weinstein, DB and JG Heider. Antiatherogenic properties of calcium antagonists. *Am J Cardiol* 59(3):163B-172B,1987.

[15] Weinstein, DB and JG Heider. Protective action of calcium channel antagonists in atherogenesis and experimental vascular injury. *Am J Hypertens* 2(3 Pt 1):205-12,1989.

[16] Davies, PF, A Robotewskyj, ML Griem, RO Dull, and DC Polacek. Hemodynamic forces and vascular cell communication in arteries. *Arch Pathol Lab Med* 116(12):1301-6,1992.

[17] Davies, PF, KA Barbee, MV Volin, A Robotewskyj, J Chen, L Joseph, ML Griem, MN Wernick, E Jacobs, DC Polacek, N dePaola, and AI Barakat. Spatial relationships in early signaling events of flow-mediated endothelial mechanotransduction. *Annu Rev Physiol* 59:527-49,1997.

[18] Eggermont, J, D Trouet, I Carton, and B Nilius. Cellular function and control of volume-regulated anion channels. *Cell Biochem Biophys* 35(3):263-74,2001.

[19] Krick, S, O Platoshyn, M Sweeney, H Kim, and JX Yuan. Activation of K^+ channels induces apoptosis in vascular smooth muscle cells. *Am J Physiol Cell Physiol* 280(4):C970-9,2001.

In: Current Topics in Atherosclerosis Research
Editor: Yong J. Geng, pp. 147-163

ISBN 1-59454-428-X

Chapter VIII

STEM CELLS IN ATHEROSCLEROSIS

Yong-Jian Geng* and Rosalinda Madonna
The Center for Cardiovascular Biology and Atherosclerosis
Department of Internal Medicine
University of Texas Health Science Center at Houston
School of Medicine

ABSTRACT

Atherosclerosis develops when the arteries cannot repair themselves properly after injury by a variety of pro-atherogenic factors. Defined by their indefinite capacity of renewal and differentiation, stem cells contribute to vascular tissue regeneration and remodeling during the development of atherosclerosis. Vascular stem cells form the vessel network during embryonic development, and in adult tissues, they generate new vascular cells that replace damaged, aged or malfunctional ones. In atherosclerosis, there are reported abnormalities of vascular stem cells that contribute to pathological alterations, including intimal hyperplasia and impairment of fibrous cap. Atherosclerosis risk factors (e.g., hypercholesterolemia, hypertension, inflammation, diabetics, smoking, obsiety, aging, etc) have profound impacts on the potency of vascular stem cells for survival, growth and differentiation. Different clinical trials have been revealing the potential benefit of stem cell therapy for treatment of patients with atherosclerosis-associated heart disease.

Color graphics are presented at the end of the chapter.

* Correspondence concerning this article should be addressed to Professor Yong-Jian Geng, MD, PhD, the Center of Cardiovascular Biology and Atherosclerosis Research, Department of Internal Medicine, University of Texas Health Science Center at Houston, Houston, TX77030. Email: yongjian.geng@uth.tmc.edu.

Keywords: Stem Cells, Proliferation, Differentiation, Atherosclerosis, Vascular Tissue Repair

Abbreviations

ESC,	embryonic stem cells;
BM,	bone marrow;
EPC,	endothelial precursor cells;
SPC,	smooth muscle prosursor cells;
Apo-E,	apolipoprotein-E;
HIF,	hypoxia induced factor;
VEGF,	vascular endothelial cell growth factor.

Introduction

Life expectancy in the western world toward the end of the 20th century reached an average of 76 years (male, 73 years; female, 79 years) [1], and most of the healthy improvement has resulted from 49% decline in the death rate for cardiovascular disease. Data from 1973 to 1993 reveals that decrease of mortality in deaths is most apparent among young and middle-aged patients with coronary heart disease [2]. According to data from the Atherosclerosis Risk in Communities Study, such favorable trends are a result of improvements in acute treatment and secondary prevention [3]. Improved living conditions, decline of a variety of infectious disease, and the advances in diagnostic techniques and therapies represent the explanations for lengthening of life expectation.

Despite the major reduction in death rates for various forms of cardiovascular disease in the developed countries, however, cardiovascular disease remains the number one cause of death [4]. One-third of men and one-tenth of women in the United States currently develop major cardiovascular disease before the age of 60 [5]. It has been projected that by the year 2020, while there will be no doubt that steady progress in treatment be achieved, coronary heart disease and stroke will still hold first and fourth places for overall death and disability, respectively, according to the World Health Organization's list of leading causes of disability [6].

For many years, scientists and physicians have devoted great efforts to delineate the etiologic and pathophysiology behind atherosclerosis as well as to develop new medicines or therapies to prevent or reverse atherosclerotic lesion development. However, the pathogenesis of this disease remains still unknown and atherosclerosis-associated heart attack and stroke is still the top killer of human beings. The histopathological alterations of this disease occur in the arterial intima resulting in a fibromuscular hyperplasia associated with variable degrees of lipids, inflammatory cell infiltration, collective tissue formation as well as calcification. With progress of this disease, the arterial tissue may undergo encroachment on the lumen or aneurismal dilatation [7]. Although the arterial intima is the major place from which most of atherosclerotic lesions develop, particularly in early stages of atherogenesis, the arterial media may display certain abnormalities including medial cell death, calcification as well as phenotypic switch of smooth muscle cells from a contractile type into a synthetic type. Among the most characteristic, microscopically visible alterations in vascular cell morphology is the formation and accumulation of lipid-laden foam cells probably transformed from macrophages and to a less extent from smooth muscle cells.

The "response-to-injury" hypothesis represents the classical paradigm of atherogenesis, proposed by Ross and his colleagues. A variety of pro-atherosclerotic factors, such as hypercholesterolemia, hypertension, diabetes, obesity, smoking and aging, can damage the vessel wall and provoke a cellular repair response to the tissue injury. It has been for a long time believed that in the response to injury, adjacent endothelial cells expand and replace damaged endothelial cells, while smooth muscle cells in the medial layers migrate into the intima and start proliferation thereafter. However, compelling evidence from recent studies on stem cells is now challenging the traditional view about endothelial cell replacement and smooth muscle cell proliferation during the development of atherosclerosis. Investigators have now been beginning understanding the complexity of vascular cellular response to injury through stem cell research.

Rapid progress in the nascent field of stem cell biology and regenerative medicine has recently attracted great attention of both publics and scientific professionals. Recently, cardiovascular stem cell research has revealed new mechanisms underlying the development of coronary heart disease [8]. In the heart with atherosclerotic coronary disease, chronic ischemia causes progressive loss of cardiovascular cells and ultimately triggers myocardial dysfunction or heart failure. Various types of stem cells from embryonic and adult tissues have potentials for regenerating functional cardiovascular cells in the heart undergoing ischemic injury. However, native or exogenous stem cells in the ischemic hearts are exposed to various proapoptotic or cytotoxic factors. Furthermore, during repopulation and differentiation, certain numbers of newly produced cells may die by apoptosis during neocardiovascular tissue remodeling and morphogenesis. Embryonic and adult stem cells may have different life spans, as being programmed genetically to apoptosis. The endogenous and environmental factors play important roles in regulation of stem cells, including inflammatory cytokines, growth factors, surface receptors, proteolytic enzymes, mitochondrial respiration, nuclear proteins, telomerase activities, hypoxia-responding proteins, and stem cell-host cell interaction. Clarification of the molecular mechanisms may help us understand and design stem cell therapies. Research has been largely focused on the role of external stem cells in repair of the injured blood vessels and in maintenance of the integrity of the blood vessel wall as well as in regulation of the pathogenesis of atherosclerosis. This new paradigm of atherogenesis may be attributed to certain abnormalities of vascular stem cells such as the intimal hyperplasia and vascular tissue remodeling. In this chapter, we will review the putative mechanisms for stem cells participating in vascular repair during atherosclerotic lesion formation and the aging process of the arterial wall. We will outline potential pathogenic and therapeutic implications for stem cell biology and technology in atherosclerotic vascular disease.

WHAT ARE STEM CELLS?

Basic scientists and clinicians are currently working together primarily on two kinds of stem cells from animals and humans: embryonic stem cells and adult stem cells. The two types of stem cells share biological activities of a stem cell in tissue morphogenesis and post-injury repairing, albeit differing in metabolism, function and morphology. In general, stem cells differ from other kinds of somatic cells in the body. Regardless of their sources, embryonic and adult stem cells share three characteristic properties:

Stem cells are premature, undifferentiated or unspecialized. One of the fundamental properties of a stem cell is that it does not have any tissue-specific structures that allow it to perform specialized functions. A stem cell cannot work with its neighbors to pump blood through the body (like a heart muscle cell); it cannot carry molecules of oxygen through the bloodstream (like a red blood cell); and it cannot fire electrochemical signals to other cells that allow the body to move or speak (like a nerve cell). However, unspecialized stem cells can give rise to specialized cells, including heart muscle cells, blood cells, or nerve cells.

Stem cells are capable of dividing and renewing themselves for long periods. Unlike muscle cells, red blood cells, or nerve cells—which do not normally replicate themselves—stem cells may replicate many times. When cells replicate themselves many times over it is called proliferation. A starting population of stem cells that proliferates for many months in the laboratory can yield millions of cells. If the resulting cells continue to be unspecialized, like the parent stem cells, the daughter cells are said to be capable of long-term self-renewal.

Stem cells can respond to exgenous or engogenous signals by differentiation or giving rise to specialized cell types. When unspecialized stem cells give rise to specialized cells, the process is called differentiation. The signals inside and outside cells that trigger stem cell differentiation have not been yet completely identified. The internal signals are controlled by a cell's genes, which are interspersed across long strands of DNA, and carry coded instructions for all the structures and functions of a cell. The external signals for cell differentiation include chemicals secreted by other cells, physical contact with neighboring cells, and certain molecules in the microenvironment.

There are different terms currently used to describe the *stemness* or *pluripotency* of stem cells to long-term survival, growth and differentiation. Depending upon their maturity or the potenial to give rise to specialized cell types, one can define a given type of stem cells as *totipotent*, *pluripotent*, *multiopotent*, *oligopotent*, and *unipotent* cellsm, By analyzeing the behavior of the cells in the intact organism (*in vivo*), under specific laboratory conditions (*in vitro*), or after transplantation *in vivo*, for decades, investigators have established and characterize stem cell lines. For example, the fertilized egg is defined to be *totipoten*, the proxy *toti* from the Latin *totus,* meaning “entire”. The totipotent stem cells or fertilized eggs have the potential to generate all the cells and tissues that make up an *embryo* and that support embryonic development *in utero*. The fertilized egg divides and differentiates until it produces a mature organism. Most scientists use the term pluripotent to describe stem cells that can give rise to cells derived from all three embryonic germ layers—*mesoderm*, *endoderm*, and *ectoderm*. These three germ layers are essentially the embryonic source of all cells of the body (Figure 1). All of the many different kinds of specialized cells that make up the body are derived from one of these germ layers. "Pluri"—derived from the Latin *plures*—

means several or many. Thus, pluripotent cells have the potential to give rise to any type of cell, a property observed in the natural course of embryonic development and under certain laboratory conditions. Thus far, only embryonic stem cells derived from the inner mass of plastocyt are capable of producing the three layer cell types, and therefore, named pluripotent stem cells. Embryonic stem cells have been for a long time used as an *in vitro* model for cardiovascular medical research.

In general, adult stem cells have limited potency of differentiation. They are often committed to one or few types of cell types in a given tissue. *Unipotent* stem cell, a term that is usually applied to a cell in adult organisms, means that the cells in question are capable of differentiating along only one lineage. "Uni" is derived from the Latin word *unus,* which means one. Usually, embryonic stem cells have much higher potency, compared to adult stem cells that reside perhaps in many differentiated, undamaged tissues which are typically multipotent, oligopotent, or unipotent and give rise to just dozen (*multipotent*), several (*oligopotent*) or only one (*unipotent*) cell type under normal conditions. This process would allow for a steady state of self-renewal for the tissue.

There are many issues investigators want to address prior to transplantion of stem cells into damaged or diseased organs or tissues. Among them, the source, quality, and availability of stem cells should be put into consideration at first. The embryonic stem cells are the most pontent stem cells, and hold a great promise for the development of new therapy. And yet, the ethic and limited resources have limited their clinical application. However, recent advances in biotechnology have led us to better understanding of the molecular and cellular basis of stem cell growth and differentiation and the potential for using the stem cells to treat various diseases, including heart disease. In this chapter, we will focus on several fundamental issues in stem cell biology as well as potential application of embryonic stem cells in cardiovascular disease.

STEM CELLS AND PATHOGENESIS OF ATHEROSCLEROSISS

The Role of Stem Cells in the Pathogenesis of Atherosclerosis: An Extension of the "Response-to-Injury" Hypothesis

Both embryonic and adult stem cells have been used for assessment of atherosclerosis in both in vitro and in vivo systems (Table 1) for different purposes. The classic "response-to-injury" theory, advocated by Ross and colleagues [9] in early 1980s, postulates that atherogenesis represents a non-specific response to endothelial damage, which can be of a variety of forms (mechanical, hemodynamic, immunological, toxic, or metabolic such caused by homocysteine and modified low density lipoprotein (LDL). Regardless of the nature of insults, which may be chemical or physical, structural or functional, injury to the arterial wall results in alteration of endothelial cell dysfunction and the ultimate loss of the anti-thrombogenic properties of the endothelium. The atherosclerotic arterial wall shows augmented adherence of platelets and inflammatory cell infiltration. Exposure to subendothelial connective tissue and tissue factors in plaques activates platelets and promotes platelet aggregation and thrombus formation. Meanwhile, various inflammatory cytokines and growth factors such as PDGF (platelet derived growth factor) are released from the injured arterial wall then which in turn stimulate smooth muscle cells (SMC), normally resident in the arterial tunica media, to migrate into the intima, where the cells proliferate, produce extracellular matrix, and together with blood-borne leukocytes, constitute the major cellular components of the intimal lesions, i.e. atherosclerotic plaques. The SMC hyperplasia induced by the vessel injury also occurs in other pathological conditions such as post-angioplasty restenosis, in-stent stenosis, and transplant arteriopathy[10].

Although the kinetics of post-atherosclerotic arterial repair and remodeling has been well documented through last decades, the origin of the cells that participate in this repair process is less clear[11]. In the response-to-injury theory, it is believed that neointimal SMC in vascular lesions originate locally from SMC of the medial layer [12]. However, more recent data suggest that other sources of vascular cells may exist, such as those circulating or resident in tissues. Vascular cells may also derived from other types of tissue cells through a process namely *transdifferentiation.* Adult, undifferentiated stem cells are frequently released from the stem cell reservoirs present in the bodies, most actively in the bone marrow. Indeed, the attachment of circulating mononuclear cells to the luminal side of the injured artery occurs prior to the development of neointimal hyperplasia exclusively due to SMC proliferation [13]. In addition, the neointimal tissue may develop in the absence of medial cells based on a model of the medial SMC deprivation by severe injury [14]. Other studies [15,16] have also reported that the SMC hyperplasia could be prevented by blocking chemokines or adhesion molecules that play a crucial role in recruiting blood cells but have no effect on migration and proliferation of differentiated SMC. Finally, neointimal SMC are distinct from medial SMC in phenotype and gene-expression patterns [17].

Table 1. Stem cells used for atherosclerosis research.

Origin	Type	Model	Reference
Embryos	ESC	In vitro gene profiling	[53]
Embryos	ESC	Transgenic Atherosclerosis	[54]
Blood	EPC	Angiogenesis in Atherosclerosis	[55]
BM	SPC	Graft atherosclerosis	[56]
Blood	EPC/SPC	Aging and Atherosclerosis	[57]

New Mechanisms for Smooth Muscle Cell Accumulation in Atherosclerotic Lesions

On contrary to the conventional assumption that damaged tissues are repaired by local parenchymal cells, a great wealth of evidence indicates the existence of somatic stem cells capable of being mobilized to remote organs, differentiate into required cell lineages, and participate in organ repair and regeneration [18-20]. Vascular stem cells may contribute to vascular repair and pathologic remodelling in models of post-angioplasty restenosis, transplant-associated arteriosclerosis and hyperlipidemia-induced atherosclerosis. A stem cell is defined by its capacity to regenerate multiple (differentiated) cell types and its ability to undergo self-renewal. In terms of commitment, progenitor cells are capable to differentiate toward particular cell lineages and have less capacity for self renewal. Studies from Asahara and colleagues in 1997 reported the existence of circulating $CD34^+$ mononuclear cells from human peripheral blood, capable to differentiate into endothelial cells in vitro, as well as incorporate at sites of angiogenesis in vivo [18]. In contrast, peripheral blood mononuclear cells seeded on the collagen nets in the presence of platelet-derived growth factor BB (PDGF-BB) transform into smooth muscle-like cells, that express alpha smooth muscle actin, myosin heavy chain, calponin and the integrins [21]. These findings indicate the existence of a common vascular progenitor cell, which can differentiate into either endothelial or smooth muscle cells (SMC) or both in the presence of lineage-specific stimuli such as vascular endothelial growth factor (VEGF) and PDGF-BB. The cytoplascity of adult stem cells challenges the traditional view that vascular progenitor cells are confined to limited vascular tissue and in the bone marrow or peripheral circulation. There is now evidence for the existence of vascular progenitor cells widely distributed throughout peripheral tissues including but not limited to the vessel wall, which can be activated in response to injury. Furthermore, in vivo studies are supporting the concept that the mature endothelium itself can generate SMC in the arteries through transdifferentiation. Vascular cell transdifferentiation (or plasticity) refers to the ability of a mature cell to acquire some or all of the characteristics of another mature cell. Two groups demonstrated that adult endothelial cells transdifferentiate into SMC in a TGF-β dependent manner [22,23]. However, only a smaller percentage (0.01 to 0.03%) of EC has been shown to be capable of differentiation or transdifferentiation. Thus, the biological significance of this finding is uncertain.

Origin of Smooth Muscle cells in Transplant Atherosclerosis

Transplant vasculopathy resembles atherosclerosis, characterized by concentric myointimal proliferation in the arteries of the graft. The neointima of the graft arteries consists of proliferating vascular smooth muscle cells and contributes to progressive occlusion of the artery, leading to down stream ischemic tissue damage and fibrosis [24,25]. Saiura et al. [26] have studied the role of bone marrow-derived stem cells in graft vasculopathy, through heterotypic cardiac transplantation between wild-type mice and ROSA26 mice, which express LacZ ubiquitously. Immunohistochemical staining with X-gal revealed that the majority of the neointima in the allograft vessels was composed of recipient cells expressing LacZ. Immunofluorescence studies revealed that *LacZ*-positive cells in the neointima expressed various markers for SMC, including myosin heavy chain, calponin, h-caldesmon and α-smooth muscle actin [14]. Conversely, when *LacZ*-positive hearts were transplanted into wild-type mice, *LacZ*-negative neointima developed on the *LacZ*-positive coronary arteries. These results indicate that the majority of the neointimal cells derived from recipient cells, but not from the medial cells of donor origin.

The identification of the source of recipient cells in the atherosclerotic allograft has been also performed by Sata et al.[14]. In their studies, the bone marrow stem cells were transplanted from *LacZ* mice to wild-type mice, and after 4 to 8 weeks wild-type hearts were transplanted into the bone marrow transplanted-wild type mice. Four weeks after cardiac transplantation, most of the neointimal cells were found LacZ positive and accumulated on the luminal side of the graft coronary arteries. Furthermore, some of the LacZ positive cells in graft vasculopathy revealed α-SMA expression. These results indicate that recipient bone marrow cells can circulate through the body and localize in atherosclerotic lesions, where they contribute to vascular remodelling and neointima formation, giving rise to both endothelial cells and SMC.

Several researchers have addressed the issue of bone marrow involvement in the process of neointimal development and SMC hyperplasia. In the studies by Schimizu and colleagues [27], a mouse aortic allotransplant model was used. In the model of bone marrow chimeric LacZ-transgenic mice, it was found that approximately 11% of neointimal SMC were of the bone marrow origin [28]. Hu et al [29] found that after vein grafting in LacZ-trangenic normal and bone marrow-chimeric mice, approximately 40% of neointimal SMC were recipient-derived whereas 60% remained donor-original. They also showed that in a similar model, large numbers of vascular cell progenitors existing in adventitia may contribute to proliferation and accumulation of intimal vascular cells [30]. However, there are some controversial reports which appear against the notion that smooth muscle cells are originated from the bone marrow. In a study on bone marrow-chimeric rats [31] the host-derived endothelial cells in advanced neointimal lesions of aortic allograft were primarily not-bone marrow derived.

Taken together, these data indicate that although the bone marrow can contribute to the population of SMC found in neointimal lesions, other non-bone marrow resources also provide precursors cells to transplanted-derived atherosclerotic lesions. Human peripheral blood has been recently shown to contain a population of circulating SMC precursor cells, and therefore it can represent a possible alternative to bone marrow in the matter of vascular progenitor cells origin. In support of this notion, data from work of Simper et al [21] show that in culture, human mononuclear blood cells can generate SMC in the presence of platelet-derived growth factor. Adipose tissue may contain precursors that may enter the vessel wall from the adventitia through vasa vasorum.

Circulating SMC precursors or progenitors might also originate from other sources, such as those from transdifferentiation of endothelial cells [32], or non-bone marrow-derived fibroblast-like cells resident in the peripheral blood [33]. In any case, it is possible that the SMC precursors can be recruited from a variety of resources depending on the severity and duration of vessel damage. If limited vessel damage occurs, medial SMC can migrate into the intima where they serve as a new source of neointimal SMC. More severe and prolonged vascular damage might signal in growth of SMC from adjacent vessels. Severe and time-restricted vessel damage will lead to recruitment from non-bone marrow sources, whereas similar damage over a prolonged period of time will probably need additional SMC precursors from the bone marrow.

Origin of Smooth Muscle Cells in Vascular Remodelling and Hyperlipidemia-Induced Atherosclerosis

The origin of smooth muscle cells in atherosclerotic lesions remains to be determined. Recent work by Sata and collegues [14] points to the contribution of bone marrow-derived stem cells to the pathogenesis of lesion formation after mechanical vascular injury, as well as atherosclerotic plaque formation after hyperlipidemia. In this study bone marrow of wild-type mice were replaced with that of LacZ mice. Four to eight weeks after bone marrow transplantation, a large wire was inserted into the femoral artery of mice, leading to endothelial denudation and apoptosis of SMC. X-gal staining revealed that LacZ-positive cells attached to the luminal side of the injured vessels, whereas immunofluorescent staining for SMC and endothelial markers revealed that some of bone marrow-derived LacZ cells in the neointimal lesions expressed α-SMC or CD31. These results indicate that bone marrow cells give rise to vascular cells, thereby contributing to arterial remodelling after mechanical injury.

Bone marrow transplantation from GFP mice and LacZ+ mice to 8-week-old apolipoprotein E-deficient (apoE$^{-/-}$) mice fed a western-type diet for 8 weeks showed the GFP- or *LacZ*-positive cells appeared in atherosclerotic lesions [14]. Immunofluorescence study revealed that GFP-positive cells accumulating in atherosclerotic plaques developed differentiational markers for smooth muscle in the aorta of bone marrow transplanted mice. For instance, most of the GFP-positive cells expressed markers for SM-α-actin. These results indicate that bone marrow cells give rise to SMC-like cells observed in hyperlipidemia-induced atherosclerosis plaques. Further analysis of the bone marrow cells that have the potential to generate vascular cells suggests that SMC may be derived from a hematopoietic stem cell (HSC)-enriched fraction positive for c-kit and Sca-1 but negative for Lin. 4 [14]. The c-kit and Sca-1 positive cells occur in the neointima of balloon-injected arterial wall. These findings indicate that the c-kit^{+}Sca-1^{+}Lin^{-} fraction of bone marrow cells has the potential to differentiate into either SMC or endothelial cells, thereby contributing to vascular remodelling.

Stem Cells in Vascular Tissue Repair and Angiogenesis

Impaired endothelial function is commonly believed as the result of arterial injury due to acute or chronic exposure to cardiovascular risk factors such as smoking, hypercaloric diet, elevated cholesterol, a sedentary life-style, diabetes, and high blood pressure. Therefore, several lines of evidence have been emerging, which suggests that impaired vascular repair reflects this ongoing injury, and disequilibrium between the magnitude of vascular injury and capacity of repair can lead to atherosclerosis. Little is known about the roles for stem cells in functional recovery even though some morphological studies indicate the stem cell contribution to regeneration of the arterial wall with atherosclerosis and mechanical injury. Full installation of functions of endothelium and smooth muscle is vital for the arterial wall carrying out its function. A functional defect artery could be vulnerable to atherogenic injury.

Production of vasoactive molecules, cytokines, and growth factors during atherogenesis trigger not only a paracrine effect on the adjacent arterial wall, but also an endocrine signal perceived by responsive remote tissues [34]. Local migration and proliferation of endothelial cells adjacent to the site of injury reflects the response of vessel wall to the injury or ischemia. Therefore, in virtue of endocrine function acquired by damaged tissues of vessel wall, peripheral tissues such as bone marrow start to carry out a repair process through the mobilization of vascular progenitor cells and their incorporation into the sites with injury [18,34-37]. It is of importance to identify particular cell populations from bone marrow in vascular repair. Intermediate vascular progenitor cells ($CD31^+CD45^-$) and more primitive stem cells ($CD34^+VEGF\text{-}R_2^+$), which constitute the total population of endothelial progenitor cells or EPC, sharing the property of DiI-acLDL uptaking, account for atheroprotective property of bone marrow. During ischemic injury, low PO_2 induces a factor named hypoxia-induced factor (HIF) which can activate transcriptin of vascular cell growth factor (VEGF) mRNA, resulting in increased production of this growth factor and vascular cell growth (Figure 2).

In the study by Rauscher and collegues, the distribution and engraftment of bone marrow-derived vascular progenitor cells into sites of atherosclerosis have been monitored [34]. Apolipoprotein-E (ApoE) deficient mice (i.e. a murine model that develops severe atherosclerosis and high cholesterol levels) were used in these experiments, where the autors investigated the effects and distributions of injected bone marrow cells in the disease process. Investigators injected bone marrow cells from normal mice (10^6 cells every 2 weeks intravenously) into atherosclerosis-prone, ApoE-deficient mice over a 14-week period starting at 3 weeks of age. As a control, an equal number of atherosclerosis-prone mice were left untreated or sham treated. Results showed an accumulation of progenitors along the arterial surface, particularly along the proximal, thoracic, and abdominal aorta where atherosclerotic lesions are most pronunciated. This was not observed in animals that did not receive bone marrow cells or those at low risk of developing atherosclerosis. A majority of the engrafted marrow cells turned out to differentiate into endothelial cells. These results demonstrate that bone marrow cells are capable to home the atherosclerosis-prone regions of the aorta and to participate in the repair process. In particular, endothelial progenitor cells can provide a pool of cells that could form a cellular patch at the site of injured vessel wall.

On account of the importance for atherogenesis of loss of equilibrium between injury and repair, and thought of the role of bone marrow-derived vascular progenitor cells in vascular repair, a key issue is what are the etiologies and mechanisms leading to affect the repair capacity of the marrow cells. Rauscher, et al. first observed that with aging, the most powerful risk factor for atherosclerosis, and in presence of other risk factors, the progenitor cells originating from the marrow become incompetent resulting in loss of their capacity for repair of the arterial wall, wich in turn becomes dysfunctional and develops lesions of atherosclerosis [34]. They treated ApoE-deficient mice with intravenous injections of cells obtained from the marrow of either young (3-4 weeks of age, before any atherosclerotic lesion could be detected) or old (6 months) ApoE-deficient mice. Whereas the young ApoE-deficient bone marrow cells maintained a repair capacity that was not detectably different form that of wild-type marrow cells, the beneficial effect of old-ApoE-deficent bone marrow cells disappeared. Analysis for specific cell populations in the bone marrow from wild type, young and old ApoE-deficient mice indicated that EPCs tended to disappear in the marrow of old ApoE-deficient mice. The results indicate that aging, in the presence of an ongoing injury such as hyperlipidemia, produces more susceptibility for atherosclerosis through the progressive exhaustion of bone marrow-derived progenitor cells, in particular EPCs, with capacity for repair of the damaged arterial wall.

The existence of a strong link between cardiovascular risk factors, vascular repair and vascular progenitor cells has been documented also in human, were researchers documented that the initiation of statin therapy increases the levels of circulating endothelial progenitor cells [38-40]. Recent studies from Tepper and collegues showed that EPC from type II diabetic patients exhibit impaired proliferation, adhesion and incorporation into vascular structures, thus account for the impaired neovascularization observed in diabetics [41]. Furthermore, recently, it has been shown that circulating EPC from high-risk subjects (e.g., diabetes, hypertension, elevated serum cholesterol levels, aging, etc) are both fewer in numbers and become senescent more rapidly than those from low-risk subjects [42]. Similarly, previous studies have noted qualitative differences between EPC form patients with symptomatic coronary artery disease and those from control subjects [40]. Low levels of circulating EPC in patients with increasing cardiovascular risk could be a byproduct of a number of mechanisms. Risk factors, by modulating the levels of oxitative stress, nitric oxide activity or other endothelial physiological processes, could directly influence the mobilization or half-life of EPC. An alternative explanation is that continous endothelial damage or dysfunction leads to depletion or exhaustation of a finite supply of EPC.

In animal studies it has been documented the existence of a link between loss of repair and early phase of atherogenesis, such as vascular inflammation. Because inflammatory markers such as C-reactive protein (CRP) and interleukin-6 (IL-6) (an interleukin that regulates the production of CRP by the liver) have been shown to identify patients at risk for cardiovascular thrombolic events [43], Rauscher and collegues tested the possibility that the inflammatory process could be linked to a deficient repair process of the arterial wall due to bone marrow senescence [34]. Authors studied the levels of IL-6 in the Apo-E-deficient mice model of atherosclerosis and observed that IL-6 levels increased form wild type mice on regular chow to ApoE-deficient mice on a high-fat diet. Such increase in IL-6 paralleled the changes in total cholesterol seen in these mice and substantially decreased after administration of bone marrow cells. Interestingly, whereas marrow cells obtained from wild type mice on regular chow brought the IL-6 level to near background, marrow cells from ApoE-deficient mice on a high-fat diet were significantly less able to reduce IL-6. These data support the hypothesis that in the absence of repair cell production by the marrow (aging marrow in the presence of risk factors), inflammation molecules increase over the capacity of organism to downregulate them through a negative feedback loop, which start with the production and release of vascular progenitor cells with capacity for repair of the damaged arterial wall. Therefore, inflammatory molecules begin to recruit inflammatory cells like activated macrophages that have the potential of further increasing the injury to the artery (positive feedback loop).

Therapeutikal Implication of Vascular Progenitor Cells

Taking in consideration the classical dogma stating that atherosclerosis is a response to endothelial damage, previous treatments have focused on eliminating multiple sources of vascular injury [12,44-46]. Therefore, the novel model of atherosclerosis in which deficient vascular repair, secondary to obsolescence of bone marrow cells, is a critical determinant of disease initiation and progression [34,41,42], might inspire an alternative approach, capable to attenuate the atherosclerosis progression, even in the presence of continued vascular injury. This new therapeutic approach is based on restoration of the capacity of the marrow to produce vascular repair endothelial progenitor cells, or on administration of exogenous endothelial progenitor cells to stabilize patients in whom the arterial repair process is markedly impaired. Outsourcing of progenitor cells has been tested in children with Hurler Syndrome, a lysosomal storage disorder first discovered in 1919, characterized by accumulation of acid mucopolysaccharides in the central nervous system and peripheral tissues [47,48]. Accelerated atherosclerosis leading to myocardial infarction and heart failure represent the cause of death, which affect patients between the ages of 10 and 20 years. In patients with Hurler Syndrome, atherosclerotic process is due to mucopolysaccharide-mediated insult to the vascular walls. Administration of umbilical blood stem cells from normal children to children with Hurler Syndrome at 16 to 18 month of age produced complete normalization of physical apperance and mental level, with substantial remission of sign of overt coronary artery disease [49]. Thus, such treatment give evidence for establishment of antiatherosclerosis applications for bone marrow derived endothelial progenitor cells.

Neverteless, it is also important to take in proper consideration that disorder of the bone marrow stem cell function contributes to pathogenesis of atherosclerosis as well, through an uncontrolled migration of vascular progenitor cells into vascular lesions and their differentiation in required cell lineages (i.e. smooth muscle cells), leading to medial hyperplasia and neointima formation [14,26-29,31]. On account of this point of view, systemic or local (e.g. drug eluting stents) strategies to inhibit smooth muscle cells progenitor cells adhesion at the vascular lesion, apparently in opposition to strategies based on outsourcing of vascular repair endothelial progenitor cells, may prove beneficial.

Our recent work has shown that transendocardial injections of autologous mononuclear bone marrow cells in patients with end-stage ischemic heart disease could safely promote neovascularization and improve perfusion and myocardial contractility [50]. The relative safety of intramyocardial injections of bone marrow-derived stem cells in humans with severe heart failure points to the potential for using stem cells to improve myocardial blood flow with associated enhancement of regional and global left ventricular function [50]. In experimental animals with chronic heart failure, we demonstrated that transplanted mesenchymal stem cells from autologous bone marrow tissue can enhance circulation by generating neovascular tissue and improving collateral blood supply [51]. Using an in vitro system, we have very recently demonstrated that treatment with the cholesterol lowering drug may attenuate expression of inducible nitric oxide synthase, a key enzyme responsible for inflammation and regulation of cell apoptosis. [52]

Conclusions

Stem cells play a critical role in tissue generation and regeneration. Embryonic stem cells can be used as an in vitro model to characterize the cellular and molecular pathways that regulate vascular cell progenitor growth and differentiation. In adults, many tissues contain stem cell-like cells, so called progenitors. In the bone marrow, blood, and connective tissue such as fat tissue, there are resting vascular cells residing and waiting for signals of activation and proliferation. During the development of atherosclerosis, the response to injury occurs in a fashion with motivation of stem cells. However, inappropriate activation, proliferation and death of stem cells may have impacts on the pathogenic alterations in the arteries with atherosclerosis. Stem cells also provide additional opportunities to repair damaged blood vessels. In order to develop therapeutic strategies for atherosclerosis and its complication, one needs to understand the phenotype and differentiation profiles of bone marrow- or other tissue-derived vascular progenitor cells.

REFERENCES

[1] *Der Fischer Weltalmanach*. Fischertaschen buch Verlag. Frankfurt; 1996.
[2] Lenfant C. Heart research: celebration and renewal. *Circulation*. 1997;96:3822-3823.
[3] Rosamond WD, Chambless LE, Folsom AR, Cooper LS, Conwill DE, Clegg L, Wang CH, Heiss G. Trends in the incidence of myocardial infarction and in mortality due to coronary heart disease. *N Engl J Med*. 1998;339:1987-1994.
[4] National Center of Health Statistics. United States, 1990. Washington, DC: U.S. Government Printing Office; 1991.
[5] Statistics NCoH. Mortality, Part A. Washington, DC; 1991.
[6] Murray JL, Lopez AD. Global burden disease study. *Lancet*. 1997;349:1269-1276.
[7] Gertz D, Kurgan A, Eisenberg D. Aneurysm of the rabbit common carotid artery induced by periarterial application of calcium chloride in vivo. *J Cin Invest*. 1988;81:649-656.
[8] Geng YJ. Molecular mechanisms for cardiovascular stem cell apoptosis and growth in the hearts with atherosclerotic coronary disease and ischemic heart failure. *Ann N Y Acad Sci*. 2003;1010:687-97.
[9] Ross R. *The pathogenesis of Atherosclerosis*. Philadelphia: Lippincott-Raven; 1996.
[10] Moore S. Pathogenesis of Atherosclerosis. *Metabolism*. 1985;Suppl 1, 34:13-16.
[11] Schwartz SM, De Blods D, O' Brien ER. The intimal soil for atherosclerosis and restenosis. *Circ Res*. 1995;77:445-465.
[12] Ross R. Atherosclerosis: an inflammatory disease. *N Engl J Med*. 1999;340:115-126.
[13] Feldman LJ, Mazighi M, Scheuble A. Differential expression of matrix metalloproteinases after stent implantation and balloon angioplasty in the hypercholestrolemic rabbit. *Circulation*. 2001;103:3117-3122.
[14] Sata M, Saiura A, Kumisato A. Hematopoietic stem cells differentiate into vascular cells that participate in the pathogenesis of atherosclerosis. *Nat Med*. 2002;8:403-409.
[15] Furukawa Y, Matsumori A, Ohashi N. Anti-monocyte chemoattractant protein-1/monocyte chemotactic and activating factor antibody inhibits neointimal hyperplasia in injured rat carotid arteries. *Circ Res*. 1999;84:306-314.

[16] Hayashi S, Watanabe N, Nakazawa K. Roles of P-selectin in inflammation, neointimal formation, and vascular remodelling in balloon-injured rat carotid arteries. *Circulation.* 2000;102:1710-1717.

[17] Zohlnofer D, Klein CA, Richter T. Gene expression profiling of human stent-induced neointima by cDNA array analysis of microscopic specimens retrieved by helix cutter atherectomy: detection of FK506-binding protein 12 upregulation. *Circulation.* 2001;103:1396-1402.

[18] Asahara T, Murohara T, Sullivan A. Isolation of putative progenitor endothelail cells for angiogenesis. *Science.* 1997;275:964-967.

[19] McKay R. Stem cells: hype and hope. *Nature.* 2000;406:361-364.

[20] Orlic D, Kajstura J, Chimenti S. Mobilized bone marrow cells repair the infarcted heart, improving function and survival. *Proc Natl Acad Sci USA.* 2001;98:10344-10349.

[21] Simper D, Stadboerger PG, Panetta CJ. Smooth muscle progenitor cells in human blood. *Circulation.* 2002;106:1199-1204.

[22] Frid MG, Kale VA, Stenmark KR. Mature vascular endothelium can give rise to smooth muscle cells via endothelial mesenchymal differentiation: in vitro analysis. *Circ Res.* 2002;90:1189-1196.

[23] Ishisaki A, Hayashi S, Li A-J, Imamura T. Human umbilical vein endothelium-derived cells retain potential to differentiate into smooth muscle like cells. *J Biol Chem.* 2003;278:1303-1309.

[24] Orosz CG, Pelletier RP. Chronic remodelling pathology in grafts. *Curr Opin Immunol.* 1997;9:676-680.

[25] Billingham ME. Cardiac transplant atherosclerosis. *Transplant Proc.* 1987;19:19-25.

[26] Saiura A, Sata M, Hirata Y. Circulating smooth muscle progenitor cells contribute to atherosclerosis. *Nat Med.* 2001;7:382-383.

[27] Shimizu K, Sugiyama S, Aikawa M, Fukumoto Y, Rabkin E, Libby P, Mitchell RN. Host bone-marrow cells are a source of donor intimal smooth muscle-like cells in murine aortic transplant arteriopathy. *Nat Med.* 2001;7:738-741.

[28] Li J, Han X, Jiang J, Zhong R, Williams GM, Pickering JG, Chow LH. Vascular smooth muscle cells of recipient origin mediate intimal expansion after aortic allotranplantation in mice. *Am J Pathol.* 2001;158:1943-1947.

[29] Hu Y, Mayr M, Metzler B, Erdel M, Davison F, Xu Q. Both donor and recipient origins of smooth muscle cells in vein graft atherosclerotic lesions. *Circ Res.* 2002;91:e13-e20.

[30] Hu Y, Zhang Z, Torsney E, Afzal AR, Davison F, Metzler B, Xu Q. Abundant progenitor cells in the adventitia contribute to atherosclerosis of vein grafts in ApoE-deficient mice. *J Clin Invest.* 2004;113:1258-65.

[31] Hillebrands JL, Klatter FA, van Dijk WD, Rozing J. The bone marrow does nor contribute substantially to host-derived endothelial cells replacement in transplant arteriosclerosis. *Nat Med.* 2002;8:2-3.

[32] Gittenberger-de Groot AC, DeRuiter MC, Berwerff M, Poelmann RE. Smooth muscle cell origin and its relation to heterogeneity in development and disease. Arterioscler Thromb *Vasc Biol.* 1999;19:1589-1594.

[33] Bucala R, Spiegel LA, Chesney J, Hogan M, Cerami A. Circulating fibrocytes define a new leukocyte subpopulation that mediates tissue repair. *Mol Med.* 1994;1:71-81.

[34] Rauscher FM, Goldschmidt-Clermont PJ, Davis BH. Aging, progenitor cells exhaustion and atherosclerosis. *Circulation.* 2003;108:457-463.

[35] Rafii S. Circulating endothelial precursors: mistery, reality and promise. *J Cin Invest.* 2000;105:17-19.

[36] Patterson C. The Ponzo effect: endothelial progenitor cells appear on the horizont. *Circulation.* 2003;107:2995-2997.

[37] Hristov M, Erl W, Weber PC. Endothelial progenitor cells: mobilization, differentiation and homing. *Arterioscler Thromb Vasc Biol.* 2003;23:1185-1189.

[38] Llevadot J, Murasawa S, Kureishi Y. HMG-CoA reductase inhibitor mobilizes bone marrow-derived endothelial progenitor cells. *J Cin Invest.* 2001;108:399-405.

[39] Dimmeler S, Aicher A, Vasa M. HMG-CoA reductase inhibitors (statins) increase endothelial progenitor cells via the PI3-kinase/Akt pathway. *J Cin Invest.* 2001;108:391-397.

[40] Vasa M, Fichtlscherer S, Adler K. Increase in circulating endothelial progenitor cells by statin therapy in patients with stable coronary artery disease. *Circulation.* 2001;103:2885-2890.

[41] Tepper OM, Galiano RD, Capla JM, Kalka C, Gagne PJ, Jacobowitz GR, Levine JP, Gurtner GC. Human endothelial progenitor cells from type II diabetics exhibit impaired proliferation, adhesion and incorporation into vascular structures. *Circulation.* 2002;106:2781-2786.

[42] Hill JM, Zalos G, Halcox JPJ, Schenke WH, Waclawiw MA, Quyyumi AA, Finkel T. Circulating endothelial progenitor cells, vascular function and cardiovascular risk. *N Engl J Med.* 2003;348:593-600.

[43] Ridker PM. Clinical application of C-reactive protein for cardiovascular disease detection and prevention. *Circulation.* 2003;107:363-369.

[44] Lusis AJ. Atherosclerosis. *Nature.* 2000;407:233-241.

[45] Boisvert WA, Spangenberg J, Curtiss LK. Treatment of severe hypercholestrolemia in apolipoprotein E-deficient mice by bonemarrow transplantation. *J Cin Invest.* 1995;96:1118-1124.

[46] Linton MF, Atkinson JB, Fazio S. Prevention of atherosclerosis in apolipoprtein E-deficient mice by bone marrow transplantation. *Science.* 1995;267:1034-1037.

[47] Hurler G. Uber einen typ multiper Abartungen, vorwiegend am Skelettsystem. *Zeitschrift fur Kinderheilkunde.* 1919;24:220-234.

[48] Dorfman A, Matalon R. The Hurler and Hunter syndromes. *Am J Pathol.* 1969;47:691-707.

[49] Peters C, Balthazor M, Shapiro EG. Outcome of unrelated donor bone marrow transplantation in 40 children with Hurler syndrome. *Blood.* 1996;87:4894-4892.

[50] Perin EC, Dohmann HF, Borojevic R, Silva SA, Sousa AL, Mesquita CT, Rossi MI, Carvalho AC, Dutra HS, Dohmann HJ, Silva GV, Belem L, Vivacqua R, Rangel FO, Esporcatte R, Geng YJ, Vaughn WK, Assad JA, Mesquita ET, Willerson JT. Transendocardial, autologous bone marrow cell transplantation for severe, chronic ischemic heart failure. *Circulation.* 2003;107:2294-302.

[51] Silva GV, Litovsky S, Assad JA, Sousa AL, Martin BJ, Vela D, Coulter SC, Lin J, Ober J, Vaughn WK, Branco RV, Oliveira EM, He R, Geng YJ, Willerson JT, Perin EC. Mesenchymal stem cells differentiate into an endothelial phenotype, enhance vascular density, and improve heart function in a canine chronic ischemia model. *Circulation.* 2005;111:150-6.

[52] Madonna R, Di Napoli P, Massaro M, Grilli A, Felaco M, De Caterina A, Daming T, De Caterina R, Geng YJ. Simvastatin attenuates expression of cytokine-inducible nitric oxide synthase in embryonic cardiac myoblasts. *J Biol Chem.* 2005.

[53] Lindmark H, Rosengren B, Hurt-Camejo E, Bruder CE. Gene expression profiling shows that macrophages derived from mouse embryonic stem cells is an improved in vitro model for studies of vascular disease. *Exp Cell Res.* 2004;300:335-44.

[54] Breslow JL. Transgenic mouse models of lipoprotein metabolism and atherosclerosis. *Proc Natl Acad Sci U S A.* 1993;90:8314-8.

[55] Xu Q, Zhang Z, Davison F, Hu Y. Circulating progenitor cells regenerate endothelium of vein graft atherosclerosis, which is diminished in ApoE-deficient mice. *Circ Res.* 2003;93:e76-86.

[56] Shimizu K, Mitchell RN. Stem cell origins of intimal cells in graft arterial disease. *Curr Atheroscler Rep.* 2003;5:230-7.

[57] Rauscher FM, Goldschmidt-Clermont PJ, Davis BH, Wang T, Gregg D, Ramaswami P, Pippen AM, Annex BH, Dong C, Taylor DA. Aging, progenitor cell exhaustion, and atherosclerosis. *Circulation.* 2003;108:457-63.

ACKNOWLEDGMENTS

This work was supported by grants to Dr. Yong-Jian Geng from the National Institutes of Health (R01HL59249 and R01HL69509), the T5 program of US Army, and Texas Higher Education Co-ordination Boards.

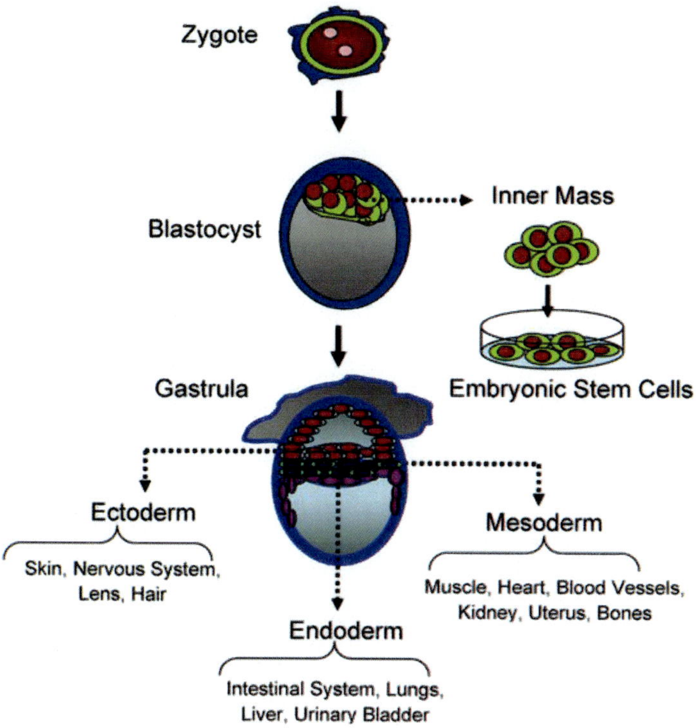

Figure 1. Schematic presentation of embryonic development of three derm layers and stem cell origin from blastocyst.

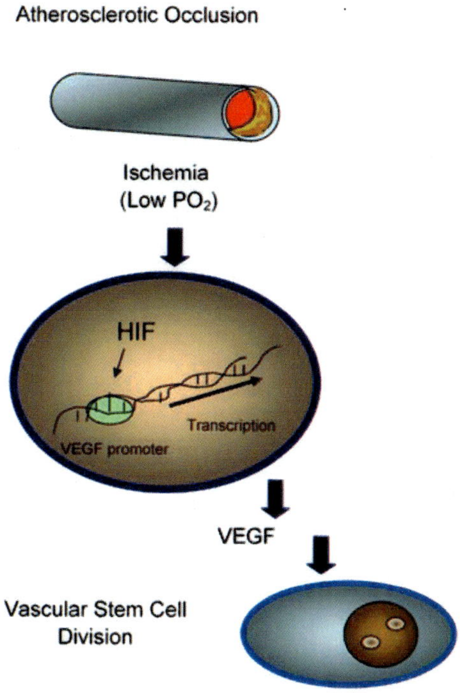

Figure 2. Atherosclerosis activates growth factor expression through ischemia-hypoxia triggered the HIF-VEGF pathway.

INDEX

A

D

E

F

G

H

I

K

L

M

N

O

P

T

U

V

W

Y